Diabetic Eye Disease

Publisher: Caroline Makepeace
Desk editor: Deena Burgess
Production controller: Chris Jarvis
Editorial assistant: Zoë A. Youd
Cover designer: Helen Brockway

DIABETIC EYE DISEASE
Identification and co-management

Edited by:

Alicja R Rudnicka

Department of Environmental and Preventive Medicine,
Wolfson Institute of Preventive Medicine,
St Bartholomew's and the Royal London School of
Medicine and Dentistry, Queen Mary and Westfield College, London, UK

Jennifer Birch

Department of Optometry and Visual Science,
City University, London, UK

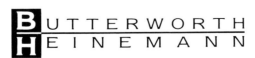

OXFORD   AUCKLAND   BOSTON   JOHANNESBURG   MELBOURNE   NEW DELHI

Butterworth-Heinemann
Linacre House, Jordan Hill, Oxford OX2 8DP
225 Wildwood Avenue, Woburn, MA 01801-2041
A division of Reed Educational and Professional Publishing Ltd

Ⓡ A member of the Reed Elsevier plc group

First published 2000

British Library Cataloguing in Publication Data
Diabetic eye disease: identification and co-management
   1. Diabetic retinopathy   2. Eye – Diseases   3. Diabetes
   I. Rudnicka, Alicja   II. Birch, Jennifer
   617.7'3

Library of Congress Cataloguing in Publication Data
Diabetic eye disease: identification and co-management/edited by Alicja R. Rudnicka,
   Jennifer Birch.
   p.; cm.
   Includes bibliographical references and index.
   ISBN 0 7506 3781 1
   1. Diabetic retinopathy.   I. Rudnicka, Alicja R.   II. Birch, Jennifer.
   [DNLM: 1. Diabetic Retinopathy – diagnosis.   2. Diabetic Retinopathy – therapy.
   WK 835 D53498
   RE661.D5 D47
   617.7'1–dc21   99–044005

ISBN 0 7506 3781 1

Composition by Genesis Typesetting, Rochester, Kent
Printed and bound in Spain

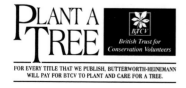

Contents

Contributors

G. W. Aylward MB BChir FRCS FRCOphth MD
*Consultant Vitreoretinal Surgeon, Moorfields
Eye Hospital, London, UK*

Jennifer Birch MPhil FCOptom DIC SMSA
*Department of Optometry and Visual Science,
City University, London, UK*

Usha Dhanesha PhD MCOptom
*Principal Optometrist, Walsgrave NHS Trust,
Coventry, UK*

Peter Hamilton FRCS FRCOphth
*Consultant Ophthalmic Surgeon, Moorfields
Eye Hospital, London, UK*

John G. Lawrenson PhD MCOptom
*Reader, Department of Optometry and Visual
Science, City University, London*

Richard Newsom MD FRCOphth
*Vitreoretinal Fellow, Southampton Eye Unit,
Southampton General Hospital,
Southampton, UK*

Christopher G. Owen PhD MCOptom
*Department of Public Health Sciences,
St George's Hospital Medical School,
London, UK*

Sarah L. Owens MD
*Associate Specialist, Retinal Diagnostic
Department, Moorfields Eye Hospital,
London, UK*

Vinod Patel MD FRCP MRCGP
*Honorary Senior Lecturer in Medicine,
University of Warwick
Consultant Physician, Endocrinology and
Diabetes, Diabetes and Endocrinology Centre,
George Eliot Hospital, Nuneaton, UK*

Alicja Rudnicka PhD MSc MCOptom
*Department of Environmental and
Preventive Medicine,
Wolfson Institute of Preventive Medicine,
London, UK*

Sailesh Sankaranarayanan MRCP MBBS
*Research Fellow in Endocrinology and
Diabetes, University of Warwick,
Honorary Registrar in Endocrinology and
Diabetes, Diabetes and Endocrinology Centre,
George Eliot Hospital, Nuneaton, UK*

Moe T. Sein MRCP MBChB
*Specialist Registrar in Medicine, Diabetes and
Endocrinology Centre, George Eliot Hospital,
Nuneaton, UK*

Paul Sullivan MB BS MD FRCOphth
*Consultant Ophthalmologist, Moorfields Eye
Hospital, London, UK*

Gillian C. Vafidis MA FRCS FRCOphth
*Consultant Ophthalmologist,
Central Eye Service,
North West London Hospitals NHS Trust*

William Vineall MA
*Camden and Islington Health Authority,
London, UK*

Preface

This book is directed towards optometrists, general practitioners, specialist registrars in general internal medicine/diabetes and doctors who may be training for their ophthalmology examinations as well as other health care professionals with an interest in identification and co-management of diabetic eye disease. Medical students requiring in-depth knowledge of the clinical and histopathological interplay between diabetes and diabetic eye disease would find this text useful. It begins with an introductory chapter into the natural history, clinical presentation, treatment and complications associated with diabetes mellitus. This is followed by a chapter emphasizing the importance of pre-conceptual advice and the clinical risk factors in the progression of diabetic retinopathy in pregnancy. Histopathology, pathogenesis and biochemical mechanisms of diabetes mellitus are described in Chapter 3 with attention to the retinal microvasculature. Findings from some of the most important epidemiology studies into the natural history of diabetic eye disease (Chapter 4) and its clinical presentation are described in detail (Chapter 5). Colour plates supported by schematic diagrams cover the spectrum of retinal features observed in diabetic retinopathy. Chapter 6 discusses the management of diabetic retinopathy and the urgency of referral for different grades of retinopathy. Recommendations laid out in Chapter 6 may need to be modified to suit locally agreed criteria for referral of diabetic retinopathy to a specialist. For the interested reader a chapter is included on the treatment for diabetic retinopathy including retinal laser photocoagulation and vitrectomy surgery (Chapter 7). Changes in visual function due to abnormalities in the retina and anterior eye in diabetes are discussed in Chapter 8.

Around 2 per cent of the UK population are believed to have diabetes, of whom approximately 200,000 have Type 1 diabetes, and more than a million have Type 2 diabetes (Calman, 1998). This has considerable implications for the management and allocation of public health funds. Diabetic retinopathy is the leading cause of blindness in people of working age in industrialized countries (Evans, 1995). It has been estimated that systematic screening for diabetic retinopathy could prevent about 260 new cases of blindness per year among people under seventy years of age in England and Wales (Rohan, Frost and Wald, 1989). Consensus is yet to be established about the most effective way to screen for sight-threatening diabetic retinopathy. Consequently there is wide variability in the screening services provided, both in coverage and methods used. Approximately 50 per cent of people with diabetes rarely or never attend hospital diabetic clinics (Gibbins and Saunders, 1989), hence, the role of general practitioners, optometrists and technicians as primary screeners has been examined. In addition, a review of patients registered blind due to diabetes in the UK revealed that 50 per cent had had no prior eye examination despite being known to have diabetes (Clark et al., 1994).

Chapter 9 explains the principles and terminology used in screening epidemiology. It reviews various screening methods that have been used to detect diabetic retinopathy. It is possible that appropriately trained and experienced optometrists, using a combined modality screening in a primary care setting, could identify with high sensitivity and specificity those patients requiring referral for treatment. It is likely that primary care-based screening will utilize one of the following, or a combination of, fundus photography with 35 mm or digital image recording and/or suitably trained optometrists performing slit-lamp biomicroscopic fundus examination (see Chapters 10, 11 and 12). The use of a recording medium has been shown in many studies to improve the sensitivity and specificity of screening for diabetic retinopathy. A recent study using a combination of measurement of visual acuity, fundus photography and direct ophthalmoscopy through dilated pupils performed by an optometrist with specialist back-up resulted in what was described as a 'fail-safe' method for detection of sight threatening retinopathy (Ryder *et al.*, 1998). The British Diabetic Association has published guidelines relating to the establishment of screening services based upon fundus photography (British Diabetic Association, 1997a) and using optometric services (British Diabetic Association, 1997b). An essential element in any diabetic retinopathy screening programme must be an efficient patient identification and re-call system. Provisions should also be made for continuing accreditation, quality assurance and audit.

Funding for screening has not yet been specifically identified on a national basis. However, classification of national screening targets and protocols is likely to form part of the National Service Framework for diabetes and is due to be published in 2001. Advice on how to approach the Health Service for support is presented in Chapter 13. An example of one scheme in operation in East London is given (Chapter 14) and it highlights the complexities encountered with the administration and documentation at each stage of the screening process.

The final chapter deals with a mixture of retinal pathologies in diabetic patients and serves as a reminder that diabetic patients can suffer ocular complications other than diabetic retinopathy.

We are very grateful to all the contributors who have worked very hard over a long time to finally make this book a reality. In particular, we would like to thank Mr Rolf Blach and Mr Peter Hamilton for initiating the co-operation between Moorfields Eye Hospital and the Department of Optometry and Visual Science at City University, which led to the formation of a diabetic co-management course for optometrists. This course was in part responsible for the genesis of this book.

Alicja R Rudnicka
Jennifer Birch

References

British Diabetic Association (1997a). Retinal photographic screening of diabetic eye disease. *British Diabetic Association Reports*. BDA.

British Diabetic Association (1997b). Optometry screening of diabetic eye disease. *British Diabetic Association Reports*. BDA.

Calman, K. (1998) On the state of the public health. *The Annual Report of the Chief Medical Officer of the Department of Health for the Year 1997*. The Stationery Office.

Clark, J. B., Grey, R. H., Lim, K. K. and Burns-Cox, C. J. (1994). Loss of vision before ophthalmic referral in blind and partially sighted diabetics in Bristol. *Br. J. Ophthalmol.*, **78**, 741–4.

Evans, J. (1995). Causes of blindness and partial sight in England and Wales 1990/91. *Studies on Medical and Population Subjects No. 57*. London, HMSO.

Gibbins, R. L. and Saunders, J. (1989). Characteristics and pattern of care of a diabetic population in mid-Wales. *J. Roy. Coll. Gen. Pract.*, **39**, 206–8.

Rohan, T. E., Frost, C. D. and Wald, N. J. (1989). Prevention of blindness by screening for diabetic retinopathy: a quantitative assessment. *Br. Med. J.*, **299**, 1198–201.

Ryder, R. E. J., Close, C. F., Krentz, A. J. *et al.* (1998). A fail-safe screening programme for diabetic retinopathy. *J. R. Coll. Physicians Lond.*, **32**, 134–7.

Chapter 1

Diabetes mellitus: the disease

Vinod Patel

Diabetes: historical perspective and introduction

A disease resembling diabetes mellitus was first described in the Ebers Papyrus from Egypt, which dates from 1550 BC. The sweet taste of urine was noted by Hindu Indian physicians in the fifth to sixth centuries AD. However, it was not until 1889 that Minkowsky and von Mering presented research showing that total pancreatectomy produced diabetes mellitus. In 1889, Laguesse named the pancreatic islets the Islets of Langerhans after their original describer. Laguesse was the first to suggest that these islets produced a hypothetical glucose-lowering substance, which was later named by Meyer in 1909 as insulin. In 1921 insulin was purified from pancreatic extracts, and hence the actual discovery of insulin is accredited to Banting, Best, Macleod and Collip. The first diabetic patient to be treated by insulin was a 14-year-old boy in early 1922 at the University of Toronto.

Diabetes mellitus continues to be an important public health problem. Although diabetes is reported to occur in 2.4 per cent of the population, it is responsible for 8.3 per cent of the NHS budget, accounting for at least £2 billion per year (*Health of the Nation*, 1994). The actual prevalence is probably much higher, with national studies from the USA showing a prevalence of 6.8 per cent in the population aged over than 19 years and 12.3 per cent in the 40–75 years age group (Harris *et al.*, 1998). The prevalence is at least 16 per cent in UK Asians over the age of 40 years (Simmons *et al.*, 1991). The number of cases of Type 2 diabetes is expected to double by the year 2010 (Zimmet and McCarthy, 1995; Zimmet and Alberti, 1997).

Clinical presentation and criteria for the diagnosis of diabetes

New criteria for the diagnosis of diabetes became necessary since blood glucose levels greater than 7.0 mmol/l are associated with diabetic retinopathy and macrovascular disease (Expert Committee on the Diagnosis and Classification of Diabetes Mellitus, 1998). Other important changes were to eliminate the terms 'insulin-dependent diabetes mellitus' (IDDM) and 'non-insulin-dependent diabetes mellitus' (NIDDM). The accepted terms are now 'Type 1' and 'Type 2' diabetes mellitus respectively, using Arabic rather than Roman numerals.

Diabetes should be considered in people with one or more of the following:

- polyuria
- polydipsia
- lethargy
- weight loss
- recurrent infections or inflammation (pruritis vulvae, balanitis, thrush, urinary tract infection)
- blurring of vision
- ulcerated feet
- poor healing
- hypertension

- ischaemic heart disease
- obesity
- family history of diabetes
- peripheral vascular disease.

Screening for diabetes mellitus should be considered in all individuals over the age of 45 years and, if normal, screening should be repeated at 3-year intervals. Consideration should also be given to screening patients at a younger age or more frequently if they are in high-risk groups. These high-risk groups include pregnant women, especially those with previous large-for-dates birthweight babies, and those over 25 years of age with one or more of the following risk factors:

- Asian origin
- a family history of diabetes
- hypertension (BP > 140/90 mmHg)
- obesity
- the elderly
- patients on long-term oral steroid treatment
- patients with a high-density lipoprotein (HDL) cholesterol level of < 1.0 mmol/l and/or a triglyceride level > 2.5 mmol/l
- those previously diagnosed as having had impaired glucose tolerance (IGT).

In the presence of symptoms, diabetes is diagnosed by a laboratory plasma venous glucose test showing ≥ 7.0 mmol/l (fasting) or ≥ 11.1 mmol/l (random). In the absence of symptoms, the test is repeated to confirm the diagnosis. The criteria for diagnosis of diabetes are summarized in Table 1.1.

A formal glucose tolerance test (GTT) is only needed in the small number of patients with borderline results from random or fasting plasma glucose testing (Table 1.2). Glucose (75 g) in water or 388 ml Lucozade™ can be used for a GTT. Only a fasting and a 2-hour sample are needed.

There is no such condition as mild diabetes. All patients who meet the criteria for diabetes mellitus are liable to the disabling long-term complications of the disease. In subjects with impaired glucose tolerance (IGT), diabetes develops in 30–50 per cent within 10 years, so screening for diabetes must be undertaken at least once a year to detect any deterioration in glucose tolerance. Stressful illnesses can result in hyperglycaemia which returns to normal but impaired glucose tolerance is often present in these patients. Urinary glycosuria allows diabetes mellitus to be considered, but is never diagnostic. Obese patients who succeed in

Table 1.1 Diagnosis of diabetes mellitus

Stage	Fasting plasma glucose (FPG) test (preferred)[1]	Random plasma glucose test	Oral glucose tolerance test (OGTT)
Diabetes (Type 1 or Type 2)	FPG ≥ 7.0 mmol/l[2]	Random plasma glucose ≥ 11.1 mmol/l plus symptoms[3]	2-hour plasma glucose ≥ 11.1 mmol/l[4]
Impaired glucose tolerance	Impaired fasting glucose (IFG) = FPG ≥ 6.1 and < 7.0 mmol/l		Impaired glucose tolerance (IGT) = 2h PG ≥ 7.8 and < 11.1 mmol/l
Normal	FPG < 6.1 mmol/l		2h PG < 7.8 mmol/l

[1] The FPG is the preferred test for diagnosis, but any one of the three listed is acceptable. In the absence of unequivocal hyperglycaemia with acute metabolic decompensation, one of these three tests should be used on a different day to confirm diagnosis. Venous plasma samples are used.

[2] Fasting is defined as no caloric intake for at least 8 hours. Water is allowed.

[3] Random = any time of the day without regard for time since last meal; symptoms are the classic ones of polyuria, polydipsia, and unexplained weight loss.

[4] OGTT should be performed using a glucose load containing the equivalent of 75 g anhydrous glucose dissolved in water or equivalent volume of Lucozade. The OGTT is not recommended for routine clinical use.

Table 1.2 Diagnosis of diabetes by the glucose tolerance test

Plasma glucose (mmol/l)	Normal	Impaired glucose tolerance	Diabetes mellitus
Fasting	4.0–6.0	6.1–6.9	≥7.0
2 hours after GTT	<7.8	≥7.8 but <11.1	≥11.1

losing weight and maintaining a lower body weight have a much lower chance of developing diabetes than those who do not lose weight. Impaired glucose tolerance is an important cardiovascular risk factor.

There is no specific drug treatment for impaired glucose tolerance. Treatment involves lifestyle management. Patients are advised to achieve or maintain their ideal body weight, take exercise, eat a healthy diet and be treated for other associated cardiovascular risk factors such as hypertension and hyperlipidaemia. The condition is important, as it is associated with significant coronary and cerebrovascular disease. IGT is not associated with the microvascular complications of diabetes (diabetic retinopathy, neuropathy and nephropathy). For insurance purposes, patients with IGT are non-diabetic.

The two main types of diabetes (Type 1 and Type 2) are described below. Worldwide malnutrition-related diabetes mellitus is common. Secondary causes of diabetes are infrequently identified in clinical practice in the UK, and include diabetes due to chronic pancreatitis, prescribed drugs, haemochromatosis, endocrine disorders (such as thyrotoxicosis, acromegaly, Cushing's syndrome, glucagonoma, phaeochromocytoma), mutant insulins and insulin-receptor abnormalities. Various syndromes are associated with diabetes, such as DIDMOAD syndrome (characterized by diabetes insipidus, diabetes mellitus optic atrophy and deafness). Gestational diabetes presents for the first time in pregnancy and often remits after delivery.

Type 1 diabetes mellitus

Type 1 diabetes mellitus was previously known as insulin-dependent diabetes mellitus (IDDM). This describes those diabetes patients who cannot survive without insulin replacement. Any patient who requires insulin treatment within the first 6 months of diagnosis of diabetes should be considered as having Type 1 diabetes mellitus. The prevalence of Type 1 diabetes in the UK is 0.20 per cent, with an annual incidence of 15/100 000 in the population aged less than 21 years. The annual incidence world-wide in the population aged less than 21 years varies from only 0.8 per 100 000 in Japan to rates of around 30 per 100 000 in Sicily and Finland. Most patients with Type 1 diabetes present before the age of 30 years, with a peak incidence at about 11–13 years of age. There is a seasonal variation, with the lowest rates in summer and spring.

In recent onset Type 1 diabetes, there is evidence of β-cell destruction with infiltration of chronic inflammatory cells ('insulitis'). This is a manifestation of continuing autoimmune β-cell destruction. Type 1 diabetes is characterized by an almost total lack of insulin due to destruction of the pancreatic β-cells. The prevalence of Type 1 diabetes is increased to 6–10 per cent in siblings of known Type 1 diabetes patients. Monozygotic twin concordance is around 50 per cent. Markers of immune β-cell destruction include islet cell autoantibodies, and autoantibodies to insulin, to glutamic acid decarboxylase and to tyrosine phosphatase. Multiple susceptibility genes (HLA DR3 DR4, DQα and β genes) have been identified which are considered essential for triggering autoimmune destruction of pancreatic β-cells (Expert Committee on the Diagnosis and Classification of Diabetes Mellitus, 1998).

The presentation is usually acute with symptoms of hyperglycaemia such as polyuria and polydipsia. Lethargy, weight loss, nausea, cramps, blurred vision and superficial infection may also herald diabetes. Nausea, vomiting and drowsiness usually occur in the setting of diabetic ketoacidosis. The acute presentation is thought to be due to the endpoint of insidious destruction of the insulin-producing β-cells of the islets of Langerhans. After starting insulin some patients experience remission; however, this is only temporary (the 'honeymoon period'). This phenomenon is probably due to the correction of hyperglycaemia, which directly damages the β-cells. The complications of diabetes (retinopathy, nephropathy and neuropathy) are uncommon before the onset of puberty, and usually present after at least 10 years duration of Type 1 diabetes. Mortality in the Type 1 diabetes patient is increased in comparison to the non-diabetic population by four- to seven-fold in the under 50 years age group.

Type 2 diabetes mellitus

Type 2 diabetes mellitus was previously known as non-insulin-dependent diabetes mellitus (NIDDM). This describes those diabetes patients who can survive without insulin replacement for at least 6 months after the diagnosis of diabetes is made. Type 2 diabetes mellitus patients can survive without treatment with exogenous insulin, although many patients with this condition eventually need insulin to improve their glycaemic control. Type 2 diabetes affects 1.2 million people in the UK, which approximates to 2.4 per cent of the population. The prevalence is much higher in the elderly and in Asians. Certain ethnic groups world-wide have a much higher prevalence; for example, the Pima Indians of Arizona have a prevalence of 50 per cent. The UK population originating from the Indian subcontinent is particularly prone to Type 2 diabetes, and this may be a consequence of the high fat, low carbohydrate, low fibre western diet or of a more affluent variation of the traditional diet.

Most Type 2 diabetics are more obese than the background population and present with insidious symptoms such as polyuria, polydipsia and blurred vision alone. They are often diagnosed incidentally in general practice after urinalysis. Type 2 diabetes is due to a combination of relative insulin deficiency and insulin resistance at the cellular level (the biological response to insulin is reduced by 40 per cent).

Insulin resistance may be promoted by obesity alone, with considerable improvement if obesity is eliminated.

The genetic predisposition to Type 2 diabetes is stronger than in Type 1 diabetes. Concordance for developing Type 1 diabetes is 30–50 per cent for identical twins, but 90–100 per cent for Type 2 diabetes. Type 2 diabetes affects at least 90 per cent of the total diabetic population and although the prevalence of the specific diabetic complications is perceived to be less than in Type 1 diabetes, the overall caseload is greater. Patterns of retinopathy may be different, with more maculopathy than proliferative disease in Type 2 diabetes. Type 2 diabetes also carries a high risk of developing macrovascular complications; strokes, coronary artery disease and peripheral vascular disease. Type 2 diabetes should certainly never be termed 'mild diabetes', particularly as the death rate is increased two- to three-fold, with a 5–10 per cent reduced life expectancy. Microvascular and macrovascular complications of diabetes are often present at diagnosis in Type 2 diabetes.

Recently, Type 2 diabetes has been regarded as conglomerate of conditions that can be considered to be a single disease. It has been given several different epithets, including Reaven's syndrome, syndrome X, metabolic syndrome and insulin resistance syndrome. The main disorders in this cluster syndrome of risk factors for macrovascular and microvascular disease are hypertension, hyperlipidaemia, insulin resistance and obesity (Reaven, 1988).

Reaven's syndrome

Type 2 diabetes mellitus should not be considered to be a disease of hyperglycaemia alone. Type 2 diabetes in most cases is better considered as syndrome X, insulin resistance syndrome or Reaven's syndrome. This comprises a metabolic syndrome that has the following four cardinal features:

1. Hyperglycaemia
2. Hypertension
3. Dyslipidaemia
4. Propensity to macrovascular disease.

Other components of syndrome X comprise increased uric acid concentration, obesity, hypertriglyceridaemia and high fibrinogen levels.

Insulin resistance syndrome has been extensively studied, but a clear clinical syndrome has not been defined. The latter in Type 2 diabetes subjects would help identify those with the highest risk of developing macrovascular and microvascular complications of diabetes. The author undertook to develop the criteria for a clinical syndrome, taking into consideration the main clinical components of Reaven's syndrome. A randomized sample of 200 Type 2 diabetes subjects from four large primary care centres was studied. The primary purpose of the study was to collect data on hypertension, lipid profile, adiposity and microalbuminuria to determine the prevalence of 'clinical Reaven's syndrome'. The latter was defined as two or more of following:

- hypertension (BP > 140/90 mmHg or on treatment for hypertension)
- dyslipidaemia (cholesterol > 5.0 mmol/l, low-density lipoprotein cholesterol (LDL) > 3.5 mmol/l, HDL < 0.9 mmol/l, triglycerides > 3.0 mmol/l)
- adiposity (BMI > 25 kg/m^2, waist/hip ratio > 0.9)
- microalbuminuria (> 30 mg/24 h).

Hypertension was present in 71.5 per cent, dyslipidaemia in 73.5 per cent, adiposity in 80.0 per cent and microalbuminuria in 8.5 per cent of subjects. Using the above definition, prevalence of clinical Reaven's syndrome was observed in 69.5 per cent of the study population. Clinical Reaven's syndrome may be a useful clinical entity to identify Type 2 diabetes patients at highest risk of developing macrovascular and microvascular complication of diabetes, and therefore allow early risk factor focused intervention.

Biochemistry of diabetes

It is now known that there are around a million islets of Langerhans, each composed of approximately 3000 cells, in the normal pancreas. These constitute only 3 per cent of the total pancreatic mass. Insulin biosynthesis proceeds through two intermediate proteins. Preproinsulin is manufactured in the endoplasmic reticulum and cleaved to proinsulin and transported to the Golgi body. The final transformation is the removal of the C peptide from the proinsulin in the Golgi apparatus. Insulin then precipitates as microcrystals in the secretory vesicles. At this stage insulin is in its final form as a 51-amino acid protein consisting of a 21 amino acid A-chain and a 30 amino acid B-chain.

An increase in the extracellular glucose concentration stimulates the release of insulin by fusion of the insulin secretory vesicles with the β-cell membrane. The release of insulin after glucose stimulation is biphasic, with a rapid first phase lasting 5–10 minutes and then a prolonged second phase lasting for the duration of the stimulus. Glucose acts via a K$^+$ channel in the β-cell membrane, the end result of which is depolarization of the membrane to allow Ca^{2+} entry into the cell and stimulate insulin release. This mechanism may explain the action of oral hypoglycaemic agents that are used to treat diabetes.

Peripherally, insulin acts on the tissues via an insulin receptor. The insulin receptor consists of two extracellular α-subunits and two transmembrane β-subunits. Insulin binding onto the α-subunit triggers a protein kinase within the β-subunit, which subsequently activates the intracellular metabolic effects of insulin. The major effect of insulin is the stimulation of nutrient uptake and biosynthetic processes. Glucose uptake is enhanced by insulin action increasing glucose transporter proteins on the cell surface. Type 2 diabetes is thought to be associated with insulin sensing and insulin-insulin receptor coupling abnormalities. Several precise abnormalities have been described, but defects identified to date only account for a very small proportion of the Type 2 population. A recently discovered feature of Type 2 diabetes is the deposition of amylin protein (37 amino acids) by the β-cells, but its role in the pathogenesis of Type 2 diabetes remains unclear.

Aim of diabetes care

The overall aim of any system of diabetes care is to produce a sustained improvement in the health experience of people with diabetes, thereby resulting in a life approaching normal expectations, both in quality and duration (British Diabetic Association, 1997). It is accepted that the maintenance of near-normal blood glucose levels is the key, not only to avoid the acute metabolic crises of hypoglycaemia and diabetic ketoacidosis, but also to prevent the development of long-term complications. Attention to cardiovascular risk factors, including smoking, hyperlipidaemia and hypertension, is essential.

Behaviour modification through education, together with regular monitoring and appropriate management of blood glucose control, is essential to the improvement of the health of people with diabetes. It is essential to remember that it is those with diabetes who play the most crucial role in this process, and hence their motivation is essential. Effective education, which is matched to their ability and capacity to learn, can enable people with diabetes to take responsibility for their own health.

People with diabetes should be empowered to obtain the maximum benefit from health care services so that, as far as possible, they are able to participate in activities open to those without diabetes. There is evidence that early detection and treatment of many established complications can reduce morbidity and healthcare costs. In retinopathy, for example, the detection of early retinal disease followed by laser treatment can prevent blindness. Planned follow-up with effective surveillance for complications is therefore essential. Management targets to reduce complications have been published by the British Diabetic Association (Table 1.3) (BDA, 1997).

Table 1.3 shows the exact targets from the *Recommendations for the Management of Diabetes in Primary Care* booklet published by the BDA. Clearly these will need to be modified extensively for individual patients according to age, general health, duration of diabetes and realism. In younger patients, stricter criteria may apply. For example, if diabetic nephropathy is present, hypertension should be treated aggressively, aiming for a BP of less than 130/85 mmHg. Shaded areas indicate local guidelines.

Table 1.3 Targets for the management of diabetes

	Good	*Acceptable*	*Poor*	*Very poor*
HbA1c%	< 6.0	6.0–7.0	7.1–8.0	> 8.0
Systolic BP (mmHg)	< 140	140–159	160–180	> 180
Diastolic BP (mmHg)	< 90	91–94	95–100	> 100
Total cholesterol (mmol/l)	< 5.2	5.2–6.4	6.5–7.8	> 7.8
Total trigs (mmol/l)	< 1.7	1.7–2.2	2.3–4.4	> 4.4
Body mass index	< 25.0	25.0–26.9	27.0–30.0	> 30.0
Fasting plasma glucose (mmol/l)	< 7.0	7.1–7.8	7.9–9.0	> 9.0

St Vincent declaration

Patients' organizations from all European countries met with diabetes experts under the aegis of the World Health Organisation and the International Diabetes Federation in St Vincent, Italy, in 1989 (Krans, 1990). Apart from a declaration on the aim of diabetes care similar to that above, targets were set for the reduction of diabetic complications. Many health authorities in the UK have adopted these as central to their diabetes care strategy. The targets are to:

- reduce the cases of new blindness due to diabetes by one-third or more
- reduce the number of people entering end-stage diabetic renal failure by at least one-third
- reduce by one-half the rate of limb amputations for diabetic gangrene
- cut morbidity and mortality from coronary heart disease in the diabetic by vigorous programmes of risk factor reduction
- achieve pregnancy outcome in the diabetic women that approximates that of non-diabetic women.

Diet and education

The impact of the diagnosis of a chronic incurable condition on a person's life should not be underestimated. It takes time for people to adjust, and patience and understanding are required from all members of the healthcare team. Education must be tailored to the individual's needs and take account of previous health beliefs and cultural differences. Objectives for diabetes education programmes have been set out by the British Diabetic Association (BDA, 1997), and the main areas that are expected to be covered are:

- an explanation of the nature of diabetes
- an explanation of the management of diabetes
- diet and diabetes
- self-monitoring
- the concept of good diabetes control
- intercurrent illness and diabetes

- hypoglycaemia
- special advice for patients on insulin
- prevention and management of long-term complications
- eye care
- foot care
- life with diabetes – the social and legal implications
- driving and diabetes
- preconception advice
- the importance of carrying identification and a warning card
- the British Diabetic Association (contact numbers).

Dietary recommendations have been set out in the BDA report entitled *Dietary Recommendations for People with Diabetes: An Update for the 1990s*. The recommended diet for people with diabetes is the diet for healthy living. This should be advocated for the whole family – not just for the patient. Patients are not being asked to go on a special diet, but rather to eat healthily. Most patients will need to make some changes to their eating habits, and the BDA recommends that all newly diagnosed patients should receive advice from a state registered dietician.

The general principles of dietary advice include the following:

1. Existing eating habits should be modified rather than an attempt made to change totally the patient's pattern of eating.
2. Total calorie intake should be restricted to that required to achieve and then maintain the agreed target body weight. About 75 per cent of people diagnosed with diabetes are overweight, and the benefits to diabetes control of approaching agreed target body weight should be stressed.
3. At least half of the dietary energy intake should be made up of carbohydrate, the majority of which should be in the form of complex carbohydrates, preferably unrefined carbohydrates with a high content of fibre (especially soluble fibre).
4. The dietary intake of refined carbohydrates, particularly sugary food and drinks, should be reduced.

5. Total fat intake should be reduced and saturated fats replaced with monounsaturated and polyunsaturated fats.
6. Dietary salt intake should be reduced.
7. Alcohol should only be consumed in moderation.
8. Special diabetic products are not necessary – they are expensive and often high in calories.

When such a diet is adhered to, many people with Type 2 diabetes become asymptomatic. Regular dietary review is vital.

Assessing glycaemic control

The HbA1c% value is the single most important laboratory investigation in diabetes care. It measures the amount of glucose covalently bonding to the haemoglobin molecule. This allows assessment of glycaemic control over the previous 60 days (half the half-life of the red blood cell). It is essential patients understand this concept and that there is an eventual aim to achieve a level of less than 7.0 per cent in the majority of diabetics. Unfortunately, the HbA1c% assay is not available for each diabetes patient at the time of assessment in a secondary care outpatient setting. This is purely due to finance, logistics and an existing culture that is reluctant to change. The current position in diabetes clinics is akin to that of a hypertension clinic measuring the blood pressure and informing the patient of the result and instigating any changes in treatment at the *next* clinic visit. Our unit has recently established a fingerprick sample postal HbA1c% service.

The fructosamine value is an index of the amount of glucose covalently bonding to serum proteins, predominantly albumin. It is a relatively cheap assay, but quality control is extremely variable, with the data being difficult to interpret. It is a measure of the glycaemic control over the preceding 14–21 days. As such it is useful in situations where meticulous control and regular monitoring is needed, for example in pregnancy and preconception care.

Both the HbA1c% and the fructosamine assay can give an erroneous indication of glycaemic control when illness affects haemoglobin or serum protein turnover. Haemoglobinopathies give erroneous glycosylated haemoglobin results. In anaemic states the glycaemic control often appears to be very good because of the increased turnover of the red blood cells. In suspicious cases haemoglobin is checked as well.

Blood glucose monitoring is relatively easy now. Strips and lancets for blood-testing devices are available on prescription. The machines are bought by the patient in most cases, but in practice have to be made available to certain special groups such as pregnant women. Lancets are less painful if used in a pricking device.

Urine monitoring can be useful if blood glucose testing is not being undertaken. Type 2 diabetic patients should do one fasting urine test and one 2 hours after a meal once a week. Urine testing in most cases should be abandoned if blood glucose is being used. Patients should seek medical advice if the fasting sample is persistently > 5 per cent.

Treatment of Type 2 diabetes mellitus

Control of the hyperglycaemia of diabetes can be achieved by various non-pharmaceutical methods, and it is extremely important to consider and promote these before using drugs. A diabetic diet with particular regard to a low refined carbohydrate, low fat and a high complex carbohydrate intake is the norm. Exercise and weight reduction also improve glycaemic control.

Oral hypoglycaemic agents are used initially, moving onto insulin therapy if the glycaemic control remains poor. Agents such as glibenclamide, tolbutamide, chlorpropamide, glipizide, gliclazide and glimepiride (all classed as sulphonylureas) stimulate the pancreatic β-cells to secrete insulin. Another commonly used agent, particularly in the obese Type 2 patient, is metformin. This is classed as a biguanide, and enhances peripheral glucose uptake and reduces the hepatic output of glucose.

Most patients can manage on diet alone, and it is good practice not to prescribe oral hypoglycaemics until the diet has been assessed and given a trial for 6–12 weeks as long as glucose levels are not persistently above 13 mmol/l. The closer a patient's body weight to the ideal, the better controlled the diabetes. Cardiovascular risk is doubled in patients with diabetes (this risk is greatly increased in diabetic nephropathy). Other preventable factors are often present and need to be dealt with to reduce overall risk (cigarette smoking, obesity, hypertension, hyperlipidaemia and lack of regular physical exercise).

Drug therapy in Type 2 diabetes mellitus

Metformin Metformin (a biguanide) works by reducing hepatic gluconeogenesis, upregulating tissue insulin receptors and thereby improving insulin resistance, promoting mild malabsorption and satiety. It is used if it proves difficult to control an overweight patient by diet alone after 6–12 weeks. It is often effective in patients without obesity. It does not cause hypoglycaemia. Long-term treatment can result in B_{12} deficiency, and this should be tested for once or twice a year. Metformin is contraindicated in patients with poor renal function (creatinine > 150 µmol/l, urea > 15 mmol/l), severe liver disease and cardiac failure because of the greatly increased risk of lactic acidosis. Metformin must be stopped in any severe intercurrent illness. The main side-effects are abdominal discomfort, nausea and loose bowel motions, particularly when treatment first starts. Taking tablets immediately prior to a meal minimizes these effects (the usual dose is 1550–2500 mg per day in divided doses).

Sulphonylureas Sulphonylureas work by stimulating insulin secretion from pancreatic β-cells. These agents are used if control is not established on diet alone after several weeks. They are often considered for first-line drug treatment in the non-obese Type 2 diabetic patient, and in addition to metformin in the obese patient. In the elderly, those drugs which have long biological half-lives and renal excretion (chlorpropamide, glibenclamide) should be avoided. Sulphonyureas, by causing hypo-glycaemia, often cause weight gain, and should only be used in obese patients following careful consideration. Warn patients of potential hypoglycaemia, particularly if alcohol is consumed. Chlorpropamide is cheap, but causes features of syndrome of inappropriate antidiuretic hormone (SIADH) in 2–5 per cent of patients and can cause prolonged hypoglycaemia. Treatment may be discontinued for these reasons. Gliclazide, a medium-acting potent sulphonylurea, has much less risk of prolonged hypoglycaemia. Some research, although not extensive, shows retardation in progression of diabetic retinopathy. Gliclazide has hepatic excretion. Glipizide is similar in action to gliclazide but with renal excretion. Tolbutamide is a short-acting sulphonylurea that is less potent than gliclazide. This is probably the safest and cheapest agent in its class, but is also inconvenient to take as it is a large tablet. Glibenclamide is a long- to medium-acting sulphonylurea and can cause severe and prolonged hypoglycaemia, particularly in elderly and renal-impaired diabetes patients. Glimepiride is a new agent with advantages of being once daily and very effective.

Acarbose Acarbose is an α-glucosidase inhibitor which reduces the absorption of glucose from the gut. Its use is limited by its side-effects of flatulence and lower abdominal pain. Some agencies consider that it should be used very early in Type 2 diabetes, as it does not promote weight gain. It is imperative that acarbose is introduced slowly and in small doses to limit side-effects.

Combination therapy The above agents are often used in combination. Metformin and a sulphonylurea are very often used together with the awareness that weight gain can be stimulated in obese patients. Acarbose can be used with any combination. Tablet treatment alone may not be appropriate when the diabetes is poorly controlled and the patient really needs insulin. Metformin is often used with insulin treatment particularly in the obese diabetic patient to improve insulin sensitivity and reduce the insulin dose.

New agents Other agents are under development. Troglitazone was the first thiazolidine-dione to be introduced, with over a million patients on this agent world-wide, especially in the USA and Japan. It has been withdrawn in the UK, however, because of its hepatic toxicity. Rosiglitazone will be licensed shortly. Repaglinide has now been approved for use, and works by closing ATP-sensitive potassium channels in pancreatic β-cells. Insulin release is plasma glucose-dependent with repaglinide.

Insulin treatment

All Type 1 diabetes patient will require insulin treatment, and at least one-third of Type 2 diabetes patients will be on insulin. Prior to the use of genetically engineered human insulin, animal insulins were used. Bovine insulin differs from human insulin by two amino acids whilst porcine insulin only differs by a single amino acid. The vast majority of patients on insulin are now on human insulin rather than animal insulin. Insulin comes in five main forms:

1. *Short-acting insulin*. This is a soluble preparation and is rapidly absorbed. Onset of action is within 30 minutes; peak action is at 1–3 h; duration of action is 4–8 h. Examples include Actrapid and Humulin S.
2. *Medium-acting insulin*. This is an isophane preparation and is less rapidly absorbed. Onset of action is within 60 minutes; peak action is at 4–6 hours; duration of action is 8–12 hours. Examples include Insulatard and Humulin I.
3. *Long-acting insulin*. This is a lente preparation with zinc and is very slowly absorbed. Onset of action is within 60 minutes; peak action is at 5–10 hours; duration of action is 24–36 hours. Examples include Humulin Zn and Ultratard.
4. *Premixed preparations of soluble and isophane insulin*. The most popular mixtures are Human Mixtard 30/70 and Humulin M3. Both of these are 30 per cent soluble and 70 per cent isophane. Other mixtures contain 10 per cent, 20 per cent, 40 per cent or 50 per cent soluble and 90 per cent, 80 per cent, 60 per cent or 50 per cent isophane respectively.
5. *Insulin analogue*. These are new, short-acting insulins. Onset of action is within 10–15 minutes, lasting for 4–5 hours only. It is used when protection from inter-meal hypoglycaemia is needed. Examples include Humalog and Novorapide.

All except the analogue and some mixtures are available in bioengineered human or animal forms (porcine or bovine). In most new cases, human insulin is used. However, existing insulin regimes should not be changed unless there are good therapeutic reasons. This is particularly to avoid hypoglycaemia, which is sometimes seen on transfer to human insulin (presumably due to the increased potency of human insulin in the presence of anti-animal insulin antibodies).

Of insulin-treated patients, 97 per cent are on either twice-daily or four times daily (sometimes termed basal-bolus) regimens. Once-daily insulin rarely produces good control.

The twice-daily insulin regime The patient injects a mixture of short- and intermediate-acting insulin in the morning (Figures 1.1, 1.2). The soluble component of the injection helps to control the hyperglycaemic effect of breakfast. During the morning, the intermediate-acting insulin begins to enter the circulation and blood glucose concentrations fall. A mid-morning snack is needed to prevent pre-lunch hypoglycaemia. Enough insulin is present at lunchtime to control the hyperglycaemic effect of that meal. Further release of intermediate-acting insulin in the afternoon necessitates a teatime snack to prevent late afternoon hypoglycaemia. The short-acting component of the evening insulin helps to control the hyperglycaemic effect of the evening meal, and the long-acting component prevents hyperglycaemia overnight. The advantage of this regime is that only two injections per day are required; the disadvantage is that lifestyle is restricted. Meals and snacks have to be of similar size and at similar

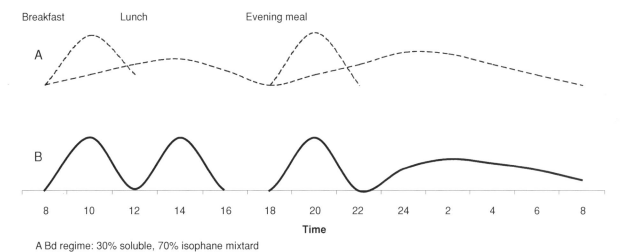

Breakfast   Lunch   Evening meal

A Bd regime: 30% soluble, 70% isophane mixtard
B Qds regime: soluble tds, overnight isophane

Figure 1.1 Commonly used insulin injections.

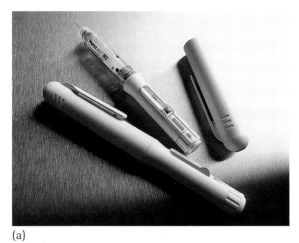

(a)

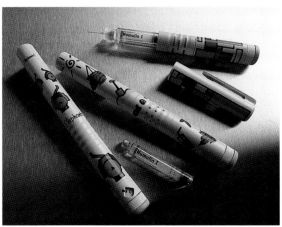

(b)

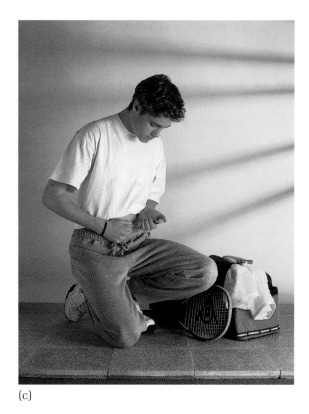

(c)

Figure 1.2 (a) and (b) Equipment for injection of insulin (pen devices). (c) Young man injecting himself.

times each day, or hypoglycaemia will result. It is almost impossible to use with shift workers or those whose mealtimes vary considerably.

Four-times daily insulin regime The patient takes an injection of soluble insulin at every meal (Figure 1.1), and the insulin helps to control the hyperglycaemic effect of the food. At bedtime a dose of intermediate-acting insulin is taken, which prevents the blood sugar gradually rising overnight. The advantage is that a more flexible lifestyle is feasible and mealtimes need not be so rigidly fixed. Size of meal can be varied at will and compensated for by varying the insulin dose, and snacks are not so essential. The disadvantage is that four injections per day are required.

Home blood glucose monitoring is very simple with the newer machines recently introduced. These enable patients to measure their blood glucose at any time of the day and adjust their insulin treatment if necessary.

Acute diabetic complications: hypoglycaemia and hyperglycaemia

All health professionals and carers dealing with diabetic patients need to be aware of hypoglycaemia. One-third of young insulin-treated patients will have a hypoglycaemic coma during their lives, and one in 10 will have a hypoglycaemic coma in any given year. Attempts to improve glycaemic control (to reduce the risk of long-term complications) appear to increase the risk of severe hypoglycaemia by at least three-fold (The Diabetes Control and Complications Trial Research Group, 1993). The main autonomic symptoms of hypoglycaemia are sweating, anxiety, tremors, feeling hot, nausea, palpitations and tingling lips. Dizziness, lethargy, confusion, difficulty in speaking, inability to concentrate and headache are caused by cerebral cortex dysfunction due to hypoglycaemia. Hunger and blurred vision are other common symptoms. The main signs are pallor, sweating, tremor, tachycardia and irritability. Focal neurological deficits may also be present and indistinguishable from stroke.

It is difficult to state an exact glucose level at which hypoglycaemia can be defined. Usually the glucose level will be less than 4 mmol/l, with profound hypoglycaemia if the level is less than 2 mmol/l.

Treatment should be started as soon as hypoglycaemia is suspected. Most cases will respond to 20 g of rapidly absorbed carbohydrate such as eight sugar cubes, four glucose tablets or 100 ml of Lucozade. This should be followed by a snack. For confused patients Hypostop gel is useful, as it can be squeezed into the mouth. Many patients in a stupor are capable of guarding their airway, and surprisingly small amounts of orally administered glucose solution given by a sympathetic attendant can wake patients sufficiently to eat their way out of hypoglycaemia. Fat delays gastric emptying, so glucose should not be given in milk. Unconscious patients not immediately responding to Hypostop will require intravenous glucose (50 ml of 50 per cent glucose). A glucagon 1 mg intramuscular injection mobilizes glucose and is often used as an adjunct. Hypoglycaemia cases due to sulphonyurea overdose or massive insulin injection require admission to hospital. On recovery, a carbohydrate-rich meal is given to prevent recurrent hypoglycaemia. The cause is established to prevent further episodes.

Hyperglycaemia is associated with diabetic keto-acidosis. In simple terms, the patient becomes under-insulinized due to lack of insulin itself or in relation to an intercurrent illness that causes insulin resistance. These illnesses include infections, trauma and myocardial infarction. Surgery may have the same effect. The basic principles of care, which must be undertaken in hospital, are to commence insulin, intravenous fluids and treatment of the underlying disorder.

Long-term complications of diabetes

The complications of diabetes can be broadly divided into microvascular and macrovascular. The macrovascular complications are responsible for 75 per cent of all deaths in diabetic patients. The most important of these is coronary artery disease, which occurs at least two to four times as often as in non-diabetic subjects (Webster and Scott, 1997). Strokes and peripheral vascular disease are also considerably more common in diabetics. Intensive treatment with insulin and improvement of glycaemic control to an HbA1c% of less than 7 per cent is associated with reduced progression of diabetic retinopathy, diabetic neuropathy, diabetic nephropathy and myocardial infarction (The Diabetes Control and Complications Trial Research Group, 1993; UK Prospective Diabetes Study Group, 1998a). Hypertension is a major treatable risk factor for almost all diabetic complications.

Hypertension

Hypertension, as defined as a BP greater than 140/90 mmHg, is present in 70 per cent of the diabetic population. Before the age of 50 years it affects 10–30 per cent of patients with Type 1 diabetes and 30–50 per cent of those with Type 2 diabetes (The Hypertension in Diabetes Study Group, 1993). Impaired glucose tolerance is also associated with hypertension (20–40 per cent).

Hypertension in diabetes is clearly associated with an increased risk of macrovascular disease – myocardial infarction, angina, strokes and peripheral vascular disease. It is also associated with an increased risk of microvascular disease. The Joint British Recommendations (1998) and the UK Prospective Diabetes Study Group (1998b) have decreed that hypertension is an important risk factor for most diabetic complications particularly stroke, death rate, heart failure, retinopathy and visual loss. Treatment should be commenced as soon as the blood pressure is greater than 140/80 mmHg, aiming for a level less than 130/80 mmHg.

General measures, such as dietary advice to lose weight, maintaining a normal salt intake, an increase in physical activity and reducing alcohol, may themselves help to reduce blood pressure. Other cardiovascular risk factors, particularly smoking and hyperlipidaemia, should also be treated energetically. First-line antihypertensive agents include ACE inhibitors, diuretics, alpha blockers and calcium channel blockers.

ACE inhibitors are highly effective except in Afro-Caribbean patients. They have also been proved to reduce urinary albumin excretion and

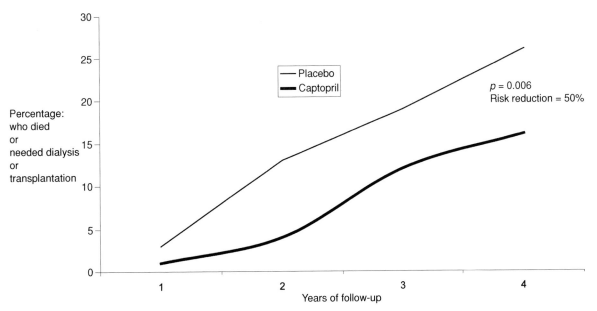

Figure 1.3 End-stage renal disease or death reduction with Captopril treatment (50 mg tds) in normotensive and hypertensive Type 1 diabetes with proteinuria.

reduce the rate of progression of diabetic nephropathy and diabetic retinopathy (Lewis *et al.*, 1993 (Figure 1.3); The EUCLID Study Group, 1997; Chaturvedi *et al.*, 1998; Patel *et al.*, 1998). There may also be a beneficial effect on cholesterol levels and insulin sensitivity. There is also a proven benefit post-myocardial infarction. A major side-effect is renal impairment, especially in patients with renal artery stenosis. It is therefore essential to check urea and electrolytes (U&Es) and creatinine and recheck them 7–10 days later. Other side-effects include hyperkalaemia and a dry cough. Drugs in this class include lisinopril, captopril, perindopril, ramipril, enalapril, fosinopril and quinapril.

Alpha blockers are extremely effective in diabetes; their main problem is postural hypotension and dizziness, particularly if diabetes has been for a long duration. There are also beneficial effects on the lipid profile with alpha blockers. Drugs in this class include doxazosin and prazosin.

Calcium channel blockers are vasodilators with no adverse metabolic effect, and may be particularly useful in patients with angina. Only long-acting agents should be used. All have some potential mild negative inotropic effect and can aggravate postural hypotension. Drugs in this class include nifedipine SR and nifedipine LA, lacidipine, amlodipine, diltiazem, verapamil and lanidipine.

Beta blockers can block insulin secretion and impair insulin sensitivity, causing hyperglycaemia, and may induce dyslipidaemia. Selective beta$_1$ agents are advantageous in that hyperglycaemic symptoms are not masked. Beta blockers are particularly useful in diabetic patients after myocardial infarction, where the benefit in improving survival after myocardial infarction is actually higher in the diabetic population than in the non-diabetic population. Drugs in this class include atenolol, metoprolol and bisoprolol.

Diuretics are very effective in diabetic hypertension, as water and sodium retention is present. However, potassium-losing diuretics can impair both insulin resistance and insulin action and therefore worsen hyperglycaemia. However, these effects are minimal with low-dose 'thiazide' diuretics, and particularly with indapamide SR. Other important side-effects include dyslipidaemia and impotence. Drugs in this class include indapamide SR, bendrofluazide, chlorthalidone and hydrochlorthiazide.

Newer agents include angiotensin II receptor antagonists, such as losartan, valsartan, candesartan and irbesartan. They are particularly useful if ACE-inhibitor side effects are pronounced. Moxonidine is a centrally-acting antihypertensive agent that is often useful.

Cardiovascular disease

Coronary heart disease (CHD) is the most common and important complication of diabetes, accounting for at least 75 per cent of deaths (Webster and Scott, 1997). There is an increased prevalence by two- to four-fold of all forms of CHD, including angina pectoris, nonfatal and fatal myocardial infarction and sudden cardiac death. Cardiac pain is often silent in diabetes because of autonomic neuropathy.

The annual mortality rate of 5.4 per cent in diabetic adults is double that of the non-diabetic population, with an overall decrease in life expectancy of 5–10 years in diabetes (Davis *et al.*, 1998). The known CHD risk factor associations in diabetes include hyperglycaemia, dyslipidaemia, increased central obesity, increased plasminogen-activator inhibitor, increased platelet aggregation, increased fibrinogen, abnormal vascular reactivity, renal dysfunction and cardiovascular autonomic neuropathy.

After myocardial infarction, in-hospital 6-month mortality rates are twice those of non-diabetic patients (Nathan *et al.*, 1997). Women with diabetes have a worse outcome than diabetic men, and Type 1 diabetes is associated with a worse outcome than Type 2 diabetes. The benefit from thrombolysis in diabetes patients is greater than in the non-diabetic population (absolute risk reduction in diabetes is 3.7 per cent versus 2.1 per cent in non-diabetic subjects) (Fibrinolytic Therapy Trialists' Collaborative Group, 1994). Outcome after cardiac surgery is slightly worse in diabetic subjects in comparison to non-diabetic subjects.

Treatment of hypertension and dyslipidaemia are important to delay the onset of CHD in diabetes. Beta blockers are under utilized in diabetic patients post-myocardial infarction, despite evidence revealing a greater treatment benefit in the diabetic in comparison to the non-diabetic population. ACE inhibitors have beneficial effects post-myocardial infarction and in cardiac failure. Hormone replacement therapy may be important in menopausal women, to afford cardiac protection after the menopause.

Strokes account for 15 per cent of all deaths in diabetes. The risk factors are almost identical to those for CHD. After a primary cerebrovascular event it is important to control for risk factors such as hypertension and dyslipidaemia. Aspirin, 75 mg daily, should be used as prophylaxis in all thrombolytic strokes and transient ischaemic attacks (TIAs), including amaurosis fugax.

Lipid disorders in diabetes

In well-controlled Type 1 diabetes, the lipid profile is similar to the non-diabetic state. In poorly controlled diabetes, triglycerides are increased, LDL cholesterol is increased and HDL cholesterol is decreased. The hypertriglyceridaemia in particular improves rapidly with insulin therapy and an improvement in glycaemic control. Type 1 patients with nephropathy develop protein abnormalities, resulting in a high LDL cholesterol even at the stage of microalbuminuria (Figure 1.4).

Lipid abnormalities occur more frequently in Type 2 diabetes than in the non-diabetic state. The characteristic dyslipidaemia is hypertriglyceridaemia, low HDL cholesterol and high LDL cholesterol (Syvanne and Taskinen, 1997). The dyslipidaemia of Type 2 diabetes is closely related to insulin resistance and hyperinsulinaemia, and is a component of syndrome X or Reaven's syndrome (glucose intolerance, hypertension, dyslipidaemia with accelerated atherosclerosis and truncal obesity).

Coronary heart disease in diabetes increases with increasing serum cholesterol levels, and the risk profile is steeper than in the non-diabetic population. Hypertriglyceridaemia is also associated with clinical macrovascular disease in diabetes. Total serum cholesterol and triglycerides should be useful for initial screening in diabetic patients once a low lipid diet has been recommended and used for 2–3 months, and a full fasting lipid profile should be checked, including total cholesterol, HDL cholesterol, LDL cholesterol and triglycerides. It is important to exclude hypothyroidism as a reason for hypercholesterolaemia.

Treatment of hyperlipidaemia includes improving glycaemic control, weight reduction and a diabetic diet. A lipid-lowering agent may be needed if target lipid parameters are not achieved. The triglyceride target is more controversial; most authorities aim for a level of < 2.3 mmol/l. After lifestyle measures, lipid-lowering agents should be considered. In diabetes, 'fibrates' are particularly useful because of their effect on hypertriglyceridaemia and hypercholesterolaemia. However, several statins are now licensed to treat hypercholesterolaemia and hypertriglyceridaemia. Moreover, following myocardial infarction the evidence is best for statins. A considerable portion of the patients in the Scandinavian Simvastatin Survival Study, WOSCOPS (5 per cent) and the CARE Study (15 per cent) had diabetes, and their expected benefit was no different or even better than in

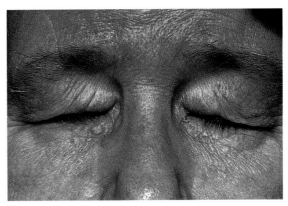

Figure 1.4 Xanthelasma hyperlipidaemia is a common complication of diabetes.

the non-diabetic subgroup (Scandinavian Sim-vastatin Survival Study Group, 1994; Shep-herd *et al.*, 1995; Sacks *et al.*, 1996). Bile acid sequestrants such as colestipol and cholestyr-amine are little used because they increase triglycerides, and because compliance is poor with these poorly tolerated medicines.

Before any drug treatment for hyperlipidae-mia is considered it must be ensured that stopping smoking, reducing obesity, reducing fat intake, increasing exercise and aspirin treatment have been advised where indi-cated.

Recent trials in cholesterol lowering treatment
In the Multiple Risk Factor Intervention Trial (MRFIT), over 360 000 men were followed up for an average of 12 years (Stamler *et al.*, 1986). There was a strong graded relationship between cholesterol level and coronary heart disease mortality. This study proved the asso-ciation between hypercholesterolaemia and coronary heart disease. The 4S (Scandinavian Simvastatin Survival Study) and the CARE Study (Cholesterol and Recurrent Events) were secondary prevention trials of simvastatin and pravastatin, respectively, in patients with myo-cardial infarction. The main findings were that with statin treatment fatal and non-fatal myo-cardial infarction were reduced by at least 25 per cent. There was a reduction in need for percutaneous transluminal coronary angio-plasty (PTCA) and coronary artery bypass surgery (CABG). Approximately 15 per cent of the trial population had diabetes in the CARE Study. WOSCOPS randomized 6595 patients with no evidence of previous myocardial infarction to pravastatin or placebo, with a 5-year follow-up. Pravastatin reduced the risk of first heart attack or coronary event by 31 per

cent, non-fatal heart attack by 31 per cent, cardiovascular death by 32 per cent, death from any cause by 22 per cent, and revascularization procedures by 37 per cent. Approximately 5 per cent of the WOSCOPS population had diabetes. It is interesting to note that pravasta-tin treatment was reported as regressing dia-betic retinopathy in a very small, uncontrolled trial (Gordan *et al.*, 1991).

The guidelines for lipid management in diabetes are shown in Table 1.4. The European Atherosclerosis Society classifies diabetes as a very high-risk category for the development of coronary heart disease. The Joint British Rec-ommendations (1998) guidelines have also been incorporated into this table.

Peripheral vascular disease

Amputation is 40 times more common in diabetic patients over the age of 65 years than in the equivalent non-diabetic population. In diabetes, because of neuropathy and arteri-opathy, the feet are extremely vulnerable to ulceration. Both peripheral neuropathy and vascular disease increase with the duration of diabetes, and are also related to smoking, glycaemic control, hypertension and dyslipi-daemia.

Various studies (e.g. Mayfield *et al.*, 1998) indicate that diabetic peripheral neuropathy is present in at least 50 per cent of diabetic patients over the age of 60 years, and at least 10–15 per cent of diabetic patients over the age of 60 years with Type 2 diabetes duration greater than 10 years have had ulceration of their feet, leading to infection. Another study showed that 7.4 per cent of diabetic patients over the age of 30 years had evidence of past or present foot ulceration, and that the prevalence

Table 1.4 Aims of lipid management in diabetes care

Total cholesterol (mmol/l)	Triglycerides (mmol/l)	HDL cholesterol (mmol/l)	LDL cholesterol (mmol/l)
< 5.0	< 2.3	> 0.9	< 3.0

of amputation was 1.3 per cent. Over the age of 70 years, 8 per cent had suffered a previous foot ulceration, with 3 per cent having had amputation (Figure 1.5).

Patients with diabetes account for 39 per cent of patients undergoing amputations, if traumatic and neoplastic amputation are excluded. The expected incidence among people with diabetes for amputation is 5.7 per 1000 patients per year. Over half the amputations were major (below and above knee, with 19 per cent having a second amputation within 3 years). The mean length of stay for a diabetic foot problem, as mentioned in the King's Fund audit, was 36.5 days.

Rates of amputation vary from 1.42 to 10.1 cases per 1000 diabetic patients per year in the UK, depending upon the accessibility and availability of a diabetic foot service. The rate in Asian patients is approximately four times *lower* than in the white Caucasian population.

Admissions for diabetic patients with peripheral vascular disease and neuropathy accounted for 20.8 per cent of the total bed days attributed to diabetes as a principal cause. Amputation receives far less attention than other complications of diabetes, and this may be due to the fact that amputation is most common among older diabetics, who tend to get less attention than the young. Clearly apathy, where it exists, is inexcusable, given the potential for reducing the amputation rate.

The way forward locally is through the development of a specialized diabetes foot team, comprising: chiropodists with a special interest in diabetes; primary care doctors with a special interest in foot care; a diabetologist; a vascular surgeon; and a radiologist.

The main aspects of clinical evaluation are:

- examination of the feet by a doctor, trained practice nurse or chiropodist at least annually, taking note of claudication, numbness, tingling or rest pain
- examination of the circulation
- examination of the peripheral pulse sensation, using vibration sense and pinprick; 10 g monofilament and neurothesimetry is useful if available
- careful examination of the interdigital areas, looking for evidence of ulceration and fungal infection
- inspection of footwear.

Feet should be examined regularly and expertly with early referral for ulcers (particularly if there is infection), as intravenous antibiotics with cover against streptococcus, staphylococcus and anaerobic organisms are often needed.

Diabetic nephropathy

Diabetic nephropathy is the commonest cause of renal failure in the UK. Diabetic nephropathy now accounts for approximately 25 per cent of all patients going onto end-stage renal replacement programmes – chronic ambulatory peritoneal dialysis (CAPD), haemodialysis and renal transplantation. Diabetic nephropathy affects 20–40 per cent of Type 1 patients and 5–10 per cent of Type 2 patients. The

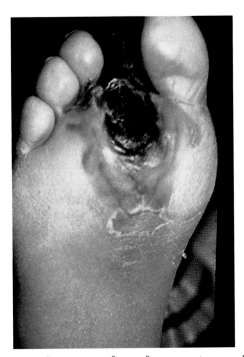

Figure 1.5 Gangrenous foot, often an outcome of poor screening for early ulceration and poor management.

incidence of diabetic nephropathy is falling, and this may be a consequence of improved diabetic control and aggressive management of hypertension. Diabetic nephropathy is heralded by persisting microalbuminuria, which is defined as an albumin excretion rate greater than 300 mg/24 h.

The natural history of diabetic nephropathy progresses from normoalbuminuria through microalbuminuria to overt proteinuria. The transition from normoalbuminuria to microalbuminuria is influenced by poor glycaemic control, hypertension, smoking and elevated HDL cholesterol. Once overt proteinuria appears (protein excretion > 300 mg/24 h), approximately 50 per cent of the patients will require some form of end-stage renal replacement programme within 10 years. The median survival from the onset of proteinuria is also 10 years. Persistent proteinuria is associated with worsening hypertension, but there is clear evidence that early effective control of blood pressure will delay progression to end-stage renal failure. All antihypertensive agents have a beneficial effect, with ACE inhibitors having the greatest effect. Recent studies indicate that the rate of decline of diabetic nephropathy to clinical states requiring renal support can be reduced by the use of specific antihypertensive agents (angiotensin-converting enzyme inhibitors such as lisinopril and captopril) (Figure 1.3) (Lewis et al., 1993; Joint National Committee on Hypertension VI, 1997). Glycaemic control and moderate protein restriction (< 0.7 g/kg of protein) may also delay progression of diabetic nephropathy.

Glomerular infiltration rate, serum creatinine and U&Es must be monitored regularly in proteinuric patients, focusing particularly on those with a duration of diabetes greater than 10 years. The interval to end-stage renal failure may be estimated by linear extrapolation plots of inverse creatinine or glomerular infiltration rate. Insulin requirements fall by 50 per cent in renal failure because of reduced renal elimination of insulin. Metformin and glibenclamide are cleared by the kidneys and can accumulate in ureamia, hyperglycaemia and, in the case of metformin, cause lactic-acidosis. These agents should therefore be discontinued and agents such as gliclazide or tolbutamide substituted.

Renal replacement therapy should be offered as freely to diabetic patients as to non-diabetic patients. Survival rates in diabetic patients receiving renal transplantation are similar to those in the non-diabetic population. The treatment of choice is renal transplantation, and this is recommended once the serum creatinine level reaches about 500–800 umol/l. The 5-year survival rate is 60 per cent for cadaver grafts, and 80 per cent for live related grafts.

Chronic haemodialysis is the most common form of treatment for diabetic patients with end-stage renal failure. However, this may be complicated by difficult vascular access, postural hypotension and poor metabolic control. The 5-year survival rate on chronic haemodialysis is 30 per cent in 45–54 year olds and 31 per cent in 55–64 year olds. Chronic ambulatory peritoneal dialysis (CAPD) is cheaper and circumvents the need for adequate vascular access. It is also suitable for older patients and those with ischaemic heart disease because of less rapid volume fluctuations. Insulin can also be added directly to the dialysis fluid, as it will be absorbed into the portal system. Peritonitis is the main complication of CAPD, but it is no more common than in non-diabetic patients. Survival is similar to that with haemodialysis.

Co-existing vascular disease, particularly retinopathy and foot problems, must be identified and treated if necessary. The major cause of death in patients with advanced diabetic nephropathy is coronary heart disease, accounting for 50–65 per cent of deaths with strokes, and peripheral vascular disease is also an important cause of morbidity and mortality.

Diabetic neuropathy

Diabetic neuropathy can be classified as reversible (painful neuropathic crises during periods of poor glycaemic control) or established (focal or multifocal, sensory or mixed). The prevalence is difficult to ascertain, as it can range from devastating crippling neuropathies to absent ankle reflexes. Wasting and painful thighs are a manifestation of diabetic amyotrophy, which often responds well to improved glycaemic control. Autonomic neuropathy results in symptoms such as postural hypotension, bladder dysfunction and erectile failure (impotence). A third nerve palsy that is painful on onset is associated with diabetes. It usually has a good outcome within 6–12 weeks.

Diabetic foot problems are almost invariably due to a combination of peripheral vascular disease and neuropathy. The pathogenic mechanisms involve both neuropathy and vasculopathy.

Erectile dysfunction has a similar aetiopathogenesis, and occurs in 30 per cent of all diabetic men and 55 per cent of those over the age of 60 years. Secondary causes also need to be considered, particularly smoking, drugs used to treat hypertension and alcohol. Hyperprolactinaemia and testosterone deficiency should be considered, but are rare causes of loss of libido and erectile dysfunction. Psychogenic causes are also likely in diabetic men and, where appropriate, referral to a psychosexual clinic may be indicated. Diabetic men with erectile dysfunction should have a detailed history and examination. Initially, the risk factors associated with impotence are assessed, particularly smoking and antihypertensive medication (beta blockade, thiazide diuretics).

The patient should then be offered information with leaflets and videos on vacuum tumescence devices and self-injection of vasoactive drugs into the corpora cavernosa or urethra (in both cases with Alprostadil E_1). An oral agent that potentiates the action of nitrous oxide (sildenafil) was recently approved for the oral treatment of erectile dysfunction. Specialized surgical referral is reserved for patients with specific anatomical problems, e.g. Peyronie's disease, arterial reconstruction and for treatment of a venous leak. Some patients may derive benefit from the insertion of malleable rods or hydraulic prostheses.

Diabetes in special groups

Diabetes in the Asian and Afro-Caribbean populations

There is now considerable evidence that the rate of diabetes in the Asian and Afro-Caribbean population is approximately three times that in the white Caucasian background population (Mather and Keen, 1985; Samanta et al., 1991). One of the major national studies was from the Foleshill ward of Coventry. This was a house-to-house survey with an oral glucose tolerance test (Simmons et al., 1991). Out of the total population found to be diabetic, 65 per cent were previously undiagnosed in the white population and 40 per cent were undiagnosed in the Asian population. Overall, the prevalence in the Asian population over the age of 70 years was 26 per cent. This is in comparison to just under 10 per cent for the Caucasian white elderly population. This study also suggested that a greater proportion of the Asian population with impaired glucose tolerance eventually go on to develop Type 2 than the white Caucasian population.

A compounding problem of diabetes in the Asian and Afro-Caribbean populations is the increased prevalence of other risk factors for microvascular and macrovascular disease, particularly hypertension. The Afro-Caribbean population has a rate of hypertension at least double that of the white Caucasian population. Screening for diabetes in Asian patients should be undertaken opportunistically, particularly when patients present with hypertension, peripheral vascular disease, ischaemic heart disease, intercurrent infection and any of the symptoms that normally suggest that diabetes should be considered.

The Hales–Barker hypothesis states that the chance of developing diabetes is increased if a small baby becomes a large adult. It is probably reasonable to suppose that first generation Asians in the UK were raised in an environment of average or below average nutrition during foetal and early development and, with later affluence and a Western diet, nutrition improved considerably to the point of overnutrition and relative insulin insufficiency.

There are also specific problems with the management of diabetes in the Asian population; for example, fasting during the month of Ramadan. This is where an absolute fast, where any food or drink is prohibited, is undertaken during the daylight hours. Insulin treatment often needs to be adjusted to avoid hypoglycaemia during the day and hyperglycaemia at night, as the main meal will be after sunset in the evening. There are also several traditional remedies for diabetes that are in use. It is difficult to discourage these, but the patient should be firmly guided by HbA1c% values as an objective measure of glycaemic control.

Diabetes in the elderly

More than half the diabetic patients are over the age of 60 years, with 95 per cent of these patients having Type 2 diabetes. Diabetes is one of the most common chronic disorders of the elderly, with a prevalence of 5–10 per cent. The elderly patient, especially if the duration of diabetes has been long, is particularly vulnerable to morbidity and mortality from hypoglycaemia and hypoglycaemia resulting in falls, injury and loss of confidence. The aims of care, dietetic advice, criteria for referral and the need for education and support of the patient are similar to those for younger patients. There are, however, points of special emphasis.

Urgent admission is required for inpatient treatment and evaluation if diabetes patients are on long-acting sulphonylureas and have hypoglycaemia, vomiting, ketonuria, uncontrollable hyperglycaemia, severe infection, pneumonia, cellulitis or a poor healing ulcer. Patients should be referred to the diabetes nurse specialist if glycaemic control is deemed to be poor. It may be possible to teach the carers the basic aspect of regular home blood glucose monitoring. Treatment should be altered if necessary, particularly avoiding long-acting sulphonylureas, such as chlorpropamide and glibenclamide. Metformin also needs to be stopped in patients with renal or hepatic impairment.

Insulin therapy is often needed, even in quite elderly patients, to relieve symptoms of hyperglycaemia, particularly lethargy, thirst, weight loss and polyuria. Once again the support of the diabetes nurse specialist can be invaluable in these circumstances to assess the home situation, assist in starting insulin and provide education and support.

Patients in residential and nursing homes are a special subgroup. Their needs are often overlooked because they are hidden in institutions and they do not fall into the normal pattern of diabetes care, with an annual review and clinical follow-up. These patients must be visited at least on a yearly basis to assess their diabetes, with particular attention to assessment of vision (cataracts and retinopathy), examination of feet, cardiac examination and renal assessment. Immobility can also lead to rapid deterioration of leg ulcers and pressure sores.

The elderly are an important consideration when diabetes care is planned, either within a practice or secondary care. This group of patients must not be neglected. Provision of chiropody and eye screening particularly needs to reach these high-risk patients.

Organization of care

The British Diabetic Association (BDA) has recently produced a leaflet for people with diabetes entitled *Diabetes Care – What You Should Expect.* The leaflet, which is available from the BDA, explains what treatment and advice patients should expect from their healthcare team. The leaflet stresses the importance of patients understanding their diabetes so that they are able to become effective members of the healthcare team. Increasingly patients will expect to receive the level of care specified in the leaflet, whether their diabetes care is being provided in a hospital or primary care setting. General practitioners have the overall responsibility for ensuring that all patients with diabetes registered on their list are involved in a planned programme of diabetes care, tailored to meet the needs of the individual patient.

The first step to achieving this aim is to identify all patients registered with the GP who have clinically diagnosed diabetes. This will involve the setting up and maintenance of a practice register of patients with diabetes, which should ideally be computerized and possibly linked to a district diabetes register. The care of patients with diabetes will, in almost every case, be a collaborative effort between a number of different health professionals, including the optometrist, practice nurse, diabetes nurse specialists, hospital diabetologist, dietician, chiropodist, out-patient nurses, local diabetes centre staff, vascular team, renal team and cardiology team. The appropriate setting for the various elements of this care will vary according to the needs of the particular patient. It will be for the GP, in consultation with the patient and members of the hospital-based diabetes team, to decide where a particular patient receives each element of care. One key aim should be the early identification and appropriate management of individuals with long-term complications of diabetes, in order to reduce:

- angina and myocardial infarction
- foot ulceration and limb amputation due to peripheral vascular disease and diabetic neuropathy
- blindness and visual impairment resulting from diabetic retinopathy
- stroke and other cerebrovascular disease
- end-stage renal failure due to diabetic nephropathy.

Strict maintenance of blood glucose control before conception and throughout pregnancy is essential in order to reduce foetal loss during pregnancy, stillbirths, congenital malformations and neonatal problems. Aspirin therapy should be considered in all diabetic patients for the prevention of cardiovascular disease (American Diabetes Association, 1998).

The annual review process is central to diabetes care in any setting. The key aspects are as follows:

1. General; discuss tobacco and alcohol, vision, driving, problems with neuropathy (including impotence), claudication, angina, shortness of breath.
2. Consider referral to a state-registered dietician with an interest in diabetes.
3. Measure weight and height; calculate body mass index and refer to a dietician if indicated.
4. Perform urinalysis for proteinuria.

5. Measure blood pressure, ideally sitting and lying, with pulse rate.
6. Assess visual acuity with a Snellen chart, with glasses if worn. If the visual acuity is less than 6/6, use a pinhole. Dilate the pupils with 0.5 per cent or 1 per cent tropicamide; Asian/Afro-Caribbean patients may require 1 per cent cyclopentolate. There is no need to screen patients under ophthalmological review or patients booked into the retinal screening programme.
7. The feet should be examined by a doctor or chiropodist (general condition of skin and nails, deformity, ulcers, peripheral pulses, vibration sense perception, pin-prick and touch). Footwear should also be examined.
8. Arrange a blood sample, ideally 2 weeks before review, for HbA1c% and creatinine (yearly at least). Measure fasting cholesterol and triglycerides every 1–3 years, depending on the last result.
9. Assess patient's knowledge of diabetes and the perception of treatment goals. Discuss management targets, with close attention to risk factors for microvascular and macrovascular complications.
10. Arrange follow-up and possible referral to optometrist, chiropodist, secondary care, retinal screening, cardiac risk clinic, vascular clinic.

Criteria for referral

The precise criteria for referral (including the timing and route) will vary between localities, and should be agreed locally. Ideally, this information should be set out in a district diabetes management policy. It is generally agreed that referral is required for the following groups of patients:

- children with diabetes – a paediatric referral is always required
- the majority of newly diagnosed patients with Type 1 diabetes
- women with diabetes who are pregnant – an urgent referral is required
- women planning a pregnancy – consider

referral for preconception advice, particularly if metabolic targets are not being met

- patients encountering problems in diabetes management, especially if agreed metabolic targets are not being met or if insulin therapy is felt necessary
- patients with protracted vomiting or keto-nuria
- patients with hypertension and/or hyper-lipidaemia if management is difficult
- patients with long-term complications:
  - persistent proteinuria
  - raised serum creatinine
  - sight-threatening retinopathy and unexplained loss of vision (see Chapter 6)
  - troublesome neuropathy, mononeuropathy, amyotrophy
  - at risk feet
  - impotence.

Prevention of diabetic complications: a strategy

1. Advice: strongly advise smoking cessation, exercise, weight reduction, adherence to diet and regularly follow-up. Stress the role of the dietician, chiropodist and diabetes care nurses. Twenty per cent of diabetic patients with severe complications will be persistent Diabetes Clinic non-attenders.
2. Screening for and effective management of early complications to reduce morbidity and mortality: hypertension, dyslipidaemia, foot ulceration, retinopathy, nephropathy.
3. Glycaemic control: aim for HbA1c% < 7.0 per cent where realistic; use metformin early in Type 2 diabetes as insulin resistance is usually present. Metformin can also be used with insulin in Type 2 patients, both as an insulin-sparing manoeuvre and to improve insulin resistance, reduce hypertension and improve lipid profile. Use multiple oral agents if needed, e.g. metformin, glimepiride/gliclazide and acarbose. Use insulin early if

HbA1c% target is not achieved. Multiple (four) insulin injections are often needed.

4. Aggressive control of any hypertension > 140/80 mmHg. If a secondary complication (particularly nephropathy) is present, aim for a BP < 130/80 mmHg. Use ACE inhibitors as first-line treatment, then diuretics (indapamide SR 1.5 mg daily may have less side-effects of hypokalaemia and insulin resistance), beta-blockers alpha blockade with doxazosin, calcium-channel blockade with a long-acting agent, angiotensin II receptor antagonists or central acting agents.
5. Post-myocardial infarction, almost all patients will need to be on aspirin and ACE inhibition. Beta blockade with atenolol, bisoprolol or metoprolol is actually more beneficial to a diabetic patient than to a non-diabetic patient. Ramipril and Lisinopril have been proven to be particularly effective in diabetic patients post-myocardial infarction.
6. All myocardial infarction and angina patients should be considered for statin Rx. Aim cholesterol < 5.0 mmol/l and LDL < 3.0 mmol/l.
7. ACE inhibitors have a special role in preventing diabetic complications. The best results in Type 1 diabetic patients with proteinuria (500 mg/24 h) are with captopril 50 mg tds. In all other groups, lisinopril 10–20 mg od has considerable evidence. Lisinopril is licensed for the treatment of hypertension in Type 2 diabetes with microalbuminuria and normotensive Type 1 diabetic patients. Diabetic retinopathy progression is also significantly halted by lisinopril in Type 1 diabetes.
8. Aspirin 75 mg od: the American Diabetes Association now advocates the use of aspirin in all diabetic patients with myocardial infarction, angina, hypertension, diabetic retinopathy and peripheral vascular disease. This simple measure is grossly under-implemented at present.

Conclusion

A major epidemic in diabetes mellitus is predicted, with all its attendant complications (Zimmet and McCarthy, 1995; Zimmet and Alberti, 1997). The management of diabetes is rewarding. With due care and attention to risk factors for diabetic complications, a considerable proportion of such complications can be delayed or avoided (Patel, 1995). At present the field of diabetes is particularly exciting, with innovative approaches to the above problems using new drugs, new screening modalities for complications and an ever larger multidisciplinary team approach. The patient with diabetes deserves our best efforts to reduce the burden of diabetes on their lives.

Acknowledgments

The author is grateful to Kamini Ganapathi for help with the manuscript and Yolanda Warren for the illustrations.

References

American Diabetes Association (1998). Aspirin therapy in diabetes. Position statement. *Clin. Diabetes*, **16**, 75–6.

British Diabetic Association (1997). *Recommendations for the Management of Diabetes in Primary Care*, 2nd edn. BDA.

Chaturvedi, N., Sijolie, A. K., Stephenson, J. M. *et al.* and the EUCLID Study Group (1998). Effect of lisinopril on progression of retinopathy in normotensive people with Type 1 diabetes. *Lancet*, **351**, 28–31.

Davis, T. M. E., Parsons, R. W., Broadhurst, R. J. *et al.* (1998). Arrhythmias and mortality after myocardial infarction in diabetic patients. *Diabetes Care*, **21**, 637–40.

Expert Committee on the Diagnosis and Classification of Diabetes Mellitus (1998). Report of the expert committee on the diagnosis and classification of diabetes mellitus. *Diabetes Care*, **21**, 5–19.

Fibrinolytic Therapy Trialists' Collaborative Group (1994). Indications for fibrinolytic therapy in suspected acute myocardial infarction: collaborative overview of early mortality and major morbidity results from all randomised trials of more than 1000 patients. *Lancet*, **343**, 311–22.

Gordan, B., Chang, S., Kavanagh, M. *et al.* (1991). The effects of lipid lowering on diabetic retinopathy. *Am. J. Ophthamol.*, **112**, 385–91.

Harris, M. I., Flegal, K. M., Cowie, C. C. *et al.* (1998). Prevalence of diabetes, impaired fasting glucose, and impaired glucose tolerance in US adults. *Diabetes Care*, **21**, 518–24.

Health of the Nation: Health Survey for England (1994). Vols 1 and 2. Department of Health, HMSO.

Joint British Recommendations on Prevention of Coronary Heart Disease in Clinical Practice (1998). *Heart*, **80** (supplement S), S1–S29.

Joint National Committee on Hypertension VI (1997). National Institute of Health 1997.

Krans, H. M. J. (ed.) (1990). *Diabetes Care and Research in Europe: St Vincent Declaration*. World Health Organisation.

Lewis, E. J., Hunsickler, L. G., Bain, R. P. and Rohde, R. D. (1993). The effect of angiotensin-converting enzyme inhibition on diabetic nephropathy. *N. Engl. J. Med.*, **329**, 1456–62.

Mather, H. M. and Keen, H. (1985). The Southall Diabetes Survey: prevalence of known diabetes in Asians and Europeans. *Br. Med. J.*, **291**, 1081–4.

Mayfield, J. A., Reiber, G. E., Sanders, L. J. *et al.* (1998). Preventive foot care in people with diabetes (technical review). *Diabetes Care*, **21**, 2161–77.

Nathan, D. M., Meigs, J. and Singer, D. E. (1997). The epidemiology of cardiovascular disease in Type 2 diabetes mellitus: how sweet it is ... or is it? *Lancet*, **350**, 4–9.

Ohkubo, Y., Kishikawa, H., Araki, E. *et al.* (1995). Intensive insulin therapy prevents the progression of diabetic microvascular complications in Japanese patients with non-insulin-dependent diabetes melllitus: a randomised prospective 6-year study. *Diabetes Res. Clin. Pract.*, **28(2)**, 103–17.

Patel, V. (1995). *Diabetic Retinopathy: Clinical and Haemodynamic Factors in the Pathogenesis*. Verlag Eul.

Patel, V. Rassam, S. M. B., Chen, H. C. *et al.* (1998). Effect of angiotension-converting enzyme inhibition with perindopril and β-blockade with atenolol on retinal blood flow in hypertensive diabetic subjects' metabolism, **47**, 12, supplement 1, 28–33.

Reaven, G. M. (1988). Role of insulin resistance in human disease. *Diabetes*, **37**, 1595–607.

Sacks, F. M., Pfeffer, M. A. and Moye, L. A. (1996). The effect of pravastatin on coronary events after myocardial infarction in patients with average cholesterol levels. *N. Engl. J. Med.*, **335**, 1001–9.

Samanta, A., Burden, A. C. and Jagger, C. (1991). A comparison of the clinical features and vascular complications of diabetes between migrant Asians and Caucasians in Leicester, UK. *Diabetes Res. Clin. Pract.*, **14**, 205–14.

Scandinavian Simvastatin Survival Study Group (1994). Randomised trial of cholesterol lowering in 4444 patients with coronary heart disease: The Scandinavian Simvastatin Survival Study (4S). *Lancet*, **344(8934)**, 1383–9.

Shepherd, J., Cobbe, S. M., Ford, I. *et al.* (1995). Prevention of coronary heart disease with pravastatin in men with hypercholesterolemia. *N. Engl. J. Med.*, **333**, 1301–7.

Simmons, D., Williams, D. R. R. and Powell, M. J. (1991). The Coventry Diabetes Study: prevalence of diabetes and impaired glucose tolerance in Europids and Asians. *Q. J. Med.*, **81(296)**, 1021–30.

Stamler, J., Wentworth, D. and Neaton, J. D. (1986). Is the relationship between serum cholesterol and risk of premature death from coronary heart disease continuous or graded? Findings in 356 222 primary screenees of the Multiple Risk Factor Intervention Trial (MRFIT). *JAMA*, **256**, 2823–8.

Syvanne, M. and Taskinen, M. R. (1997). Lipids and lipoproteins as coronary risk factors in non-insulin-dependent diabetes mellitus. *Lancet.*, **350**, 20–23.

The Diabetes Control and Complications Trial Research Group (1993). The effect of intensive treatment of diabetes on the development and progression of long-term complications in insulin-dependent diabetes mellitus. *N. Engl. J. Med.*, **329**, 977–86.

The EUCLID Study Group (1997). Randomised placebo-controlled trial of lisinopril in normotensive patients with insulin-dependent diabetes and normoalbuminuria or microalbuminuria. *Lancet*, **349**, 1787–92.

The Hypertension in Diabetes Study Group (1993). Hypertension in Diabetes study: II Increased risk of cardiovascular complications in hypertensive Type 2 diabetic patients. *J. Hypertens.*, **11**, 319–25.

UK Prospective Diabetes Study Group (1998a). Intensive blood-glucose control with sulphonylureas or insulin compared with conventional treatment and risk of complications in patients with type 2 diabetes (UKPDS 33). *Lancet*, **352**, 837–53.

UK Prospective Diabetes Study Group (1998b). Tight blood pressure control and risk of macrovascular and microvascular complications in type 2 diabetes (UKPDS 38). *Br. Med. J.*, **317**, 703–13.

Webster, M. W. I. and Scott, R. S. (1997). What cardiologists need to know about diabetes. *Lancet*, **350**, 23–8.

Zimmet, P. Z. and Alberti, K. G. M. M. (1997). The changing face of macrovascular disease in non-insulin-dependent diabetes mellitus: an epidemic in progress. *Lancet*, **350**, 1–4.

Zimmet, P. and McCarthy, D. (1995). The NIDDM epidemic: global estimates and projections – a look into the crystal ball. *IDF Bull.*, **40(3)**, 8–16.

Further reading

American Diabetes Association (2000). Clinical practice recommendations. *Diabetes Care*, **23** (supplement 1), S1–110.

Brunner, F. P., Brynger, H., Challah, S. *et al.* (1988). Renal replacement therapy in patients with diabetic nephropathy, 1980–1985. Report from the European Dialysis and Transplant Association Registry. *Nephr. Dial. Transplant*, **3**, 585–95.

Pickup, J. C. and Williams, G. (eds) (1997). *Textbook of Diabetes*, 2nd edn. Blackwell Science.

Von Engelhart, D. (1983). *Diabetes: Its Medical and Cultural History*. Springer-Verlag.

Young, M. J., Boulton, A. J. M., Macleod, A. F. *et al.* (1993). Multicentre study of the prevalence of diabetic peripheral neuropathy in the United Kingdom hospital clinic population. *Diabetologia*, **36**, 150–54.

Chapter 2

Pregnancy and diabetic retinopathy

Sailesh Sankaranarayanan, Moe T. Sein and
Vinod Patel

Introduction and clinical studies

Pregnancy has been associated with an increased progression of certain diabetic complications, particularly retinopathy and nephropathy. Studies on the effect of pregnancy on the natural history of diabetic retinopathy generally indicate a trend towards increased progression. The largest epidemiological study of the natural history of diabetic retinopathy was the Wisconsin Epidemiologic Study of Diabetic Retinopathy (WESDR). The severity of retinopathy was graded using the gold standard of seven-field colour photography (Klein *et al.*, 1990). After adjusting for the glycated haemoglobin value, current pregnancy was significantly associated with a 2.3-fold increase in progression of retinopathy compared with non-pregnant diabetic women over the same time period. The elegant fluorescein angiogram studies of Soubrane *et al.* (1985) quantified this process by microaneurysm counting. The microaneurysm counts during the course of pregnancy and post-partum were as follows: pre-pregnancy, 42.7 ± 6.9; before 28 weeks gestation, 56.7 ± 8.8; 35 weeks gestation, 79.7 ± 13.4; 6 months post-partum, 62.7 ± 10.4; >15 months post-partum, 60.3 ± 8.8 (Doubrane *et al.*, 1985).

An early study showed that the prevalence of diabetic retinopathy was 77.4 per cent in 53 pregnant diabetic women versus 46.2 per cent in 39 age-matched non-pregnant diabetic controls (Moloney and Drury, 1982). Worsening of retinopathy was reported in 16 per cent of pregnant diabetic women in comparison to 6 per cent of non-pregnant diabetic women within a similar timeframe (Ayed *et al.*, 1992). It became apparent in the early 1980s that rapid improvement in glycaemic control resulted in early short-term deterioration of diabetic retinopathy. This was confirmed in diabetic pregnancies, with diabetic retinopathy deteriorating most markedly in diabetic patients demonstrating the largest excursion between their initial poor control and subsequent good glycaemic control (Phelps *et al.*, 1986). It must be stressed that progression of retinopathy to proliferation is rare without significant pre-pregnancy diabetic retinopathy. Axer-Siegel *et al.* (1996) reported that in 65 Type 1 diabetic patients, progression of diabetic retinopathy occurred in 77.5 per cent who presented with retinopathy at conception. Progression to proliferative diabetic retinopathy occurred in 22.5 per cent. Only 26 per cent of the patients without retinopathy at the start of their pregnancy had progression of retinopathy. The clinical risk factors associated with progression of diabetic retinopathy were longer duration of diabetes, higher HbA1c%, and systolic hypertension.

The case reported by Hagay *et al.* (1994) serves to highlight two clinical points. They reported the case of a patient with gestational diabetes who had very poor glycaemic control at presentation, with an HbA1c% of 16.2 per cent. The HbA1c% or glycated haemoglobin is a measure of glucose covalently bound to the haemoglobin molecule. As it reflects an integral of the plasma glucose over the last 60 days, it is used to indicate glycaemic control. A HbA1c% value of <7 per cent shows good glycaemic control, with levels >9 per cent indicating very poor glycaemic control. In the reported case glycaemic control was improved rapidly, achieving an HbA1c% of 5.9 per cent 12 weeks later, but the patient developed severe bilateral proliferative diabetic retinopathy. This case firmly reiterates the message that glycaemic control should be improved slowly. Our practice is to have a preconception session with the diabetic patient so that excellent glycaemic control is attempted prior to conception (HbA1c% <7 per cent). Several studies have shown that good control of blood glucose levels and/or HbA1c% is associated with a lower prevalence of retinopathy (UKPDS Group, 1988; DCCT Research Group, 1993).

Excellent well-established metabolic control before conception is required to minimize the risk of progression of retinopathy. Those with moderate to severe retinopathy at conception need more careful ophthalmic monitoring, particularly if their diabetes has been suboptimally controlled (Chew et al., 1995). An increase in the rate of deterioration of visual acuity and blindness has been reported if initial proliferative retinopathy was present (Hopp et al., 1995). One study compared conventional insulin therapy with intensive insulin infusion therapy during the first trimester of pregnancy (Jovanovic-Peterson and Peterson, 1991). This showed that the proportion of patients progressing with respect to their retinopathy did not differ significantly between the groups, and in the majority the deterioration was minimal. However, two patients in the intensive therapy group developed acute ischaemic retinopathy that progressed to a proliferative stage in spite of laser treatment. In these two cases, the decrease in the HbA1c% level was among the greatest and fastest in the study. These data show that a rapid near normalization of glycaemic control by intensive insulin therapy during pregnancy can accelerate the progression of retinopathy in poorly controlled diabetic patients. Prudent practice would suggest that a pregnancy be planned to be able to normalize the blood glucose slowly (over 6–8 months) before conception (Jovanovic-Peterson and Peterson, 1991). Ideally, the aim should be an HbA1c% of <7 per cent. Once pregnancy is diagnosed, glycaemic control should improve at a rate of no more than 1 per cent HbA1c per month. There was an increased prevalence of hypertension and pre-eclampsia (hypertension, oedema, headaches) in the majority of patients with severe diabetic retinopathy or nephropathy (Jovanovic-Peterson and Peterson, 1991). Whether systolic or diastolic pressure is the more significant risk factor is still controversial.

At this stage it is important to dispel two myths about pregnancy and diabetic retinopathy. First, therapeutic abortion was previously recommended for patients with proliferative diabetic retinopathy. However, most cases respond extremely favourably to laser photocoagulation. Second, Caesarian section was deemed necessary in diabetic patients with proliferative diabetic retinopathy to reduce the chances of progression to vitreous haemorrhage. This is not necessary unless indicated for obstetric complications in the vast majority of cases.

Diabetic retinopathy: pathogenic mechanisms in pregnancy

The pathogenesis of diabetic retinopathy includes many factors, the most important of which are haemodynamic, endocrine and biochemical. Only factors relatively specific to the diabetic pregnancy need be considered. Higher serum PZ (protein Z) concentrations are significantly more frequent among pregnant diabetic patients without proliferative retinopathy (Briese et al., 1991). In contrast, the mean values in mothers with diabetes mellitus complicated by proliferative retinopathy continue to decrease. Very low levels of PZ in diabetic pregnancies have been associated with severe proliferative retinopathy. Therefore, measurement of serum PZ in diabetic pregnancy might help to predict the risk of progressive retinopathy (Briese et al., 1991). Another factor related to diabetic retinopathy is fibroblast growth factor 2 (FGF-2), which is a potent mitogen and angiogenic factor normally absent from the non-pregnant adult circulation. However, this factor is present in normal maternal serum. Immunoreactive FGF-2 is detectable at 14 weeks and reaches a maximum at 26 weeks, after which values steadily declined to term. Circulating FGF-2 levels are particularly elevated in pregnancies complicated by diabetes. Serum FGF-2 is also more abundant in pregnant diabetic women with retinopathy than in those without retinopathy.

A high circulating level of FGF-2 may be causally related to the development of diabetic retinopathy. It is also likely that elevated FGF-2 values reflect poor glycaemic control, as the FGF-2 level is positively correlated with the HbA1c% values at 22, 30 and 34 weeks gestation (Hill *et al.*, 1997).

A haemodynamic model for the pathogenesis of diabetic retinopathy in pregnancy

Pregnancy is a period of immense physiological change in the human circulation. Cardiac output increases by 40 per cent due to a combination of increased heart rate and circulatory volume together with a decreased vascular resistance. This may lead to increased retinal blood flow and may, at least in part, be responsible for the increased progression of retinopathy in the diabetic pregnancy. The haemodynamic model as applied to the general diabetic retinal circulation will be examined in detail before specifically reviewing the retinal circulation in the diabetic pregnancy.

Abnormalities of retinal blood flow and its regulation in patients with diabetes mellitus have been shown by many investigators. It has been proposed that increased retinal blood flow leading to increased shear stress on the vascular endothelium is an important pathogenic mechanism for diabetic retinopathy (Patel *et al.*, 1992). Interestingly, a rapid reduction in retinal blood flow is also associated with progression of diabetic retinopathy. Clinically, this is seen when glycaemic control is improved quickly, as in pregnancy, and when intensive glycaemic control is instituted

with multiple insulin injections or with a continuous infusion of insulin. It has now been shown in several studies that intensive insulin therapy rapidly achieving a near normal HbA1c% (< 7 per cent) is associated with a higher rate of deterioration of diabetic retinopathy, with more cotton wool spots and intraretinal microvascular abnormalities (KROC Collaborative Study Group, 1984). The Oslo Study demonstrated this phenomenon with worsening of retinopathy in the short-term, but their 7-year follow-up data showed a clear net beneficial effect of improved diabetic control with a reduced rate of progression of diabetic retinopathy (Brinchmann-Hansen *et al.*, 1992). All doubts about the importance of glycaemic control have been laid to rest with the publication of the large randomized DCCT Study (Diabetes Control and Complications Study) which studied 1441 Type 1 diabetic subjects over 6.5 years (The Diabetes Control and Complications Trial Research Group, 1993). This compared intensive treatment reducing the HbA1c% to less than 7.0 per cent with more conventional treatment and a HbA1c% level of 9 per cent. Intensive control reduced the progression of diabetic retinopathy in the primary prevention cohort by 76 per cent and in the secondary prevention cohort by 54 per cent. A rapid improvement in glycaemic control is associated with a reduction in retinal blood flow. The lesions (cotton wool spots, haemorrhages, intraretinal microvascular abnormalities) associated with a reduction in retinal blood flow are those of retinal ischaemia.

In a hyperdynamic circulation (as in pregnancy and hypertension), retinal blood flow increases in direct proportion to the perfusion pressure unless there is a protective regulatory response. This response is autoregulation, and is defined as the intrinsic myogenic ability of blood vessels to keep blood flow to a tissue bed constant in conditions of varying perfusion pressure. Autoregulation is particularly important in the human retinal circulation, as it lacks an autonomic innervation. If autoregulation fails then retinal blood flow will increase, leading to an increment in shear stress to the vessel wall since shear stress is directly proportional to flow (Milnor, 1989). Injury to the endothelium can result from shear stress alone with concomitant damage to pericyte and endothelial cells, as demonstrated in experimental hypertension (Garner et al., 1975; Tso and Jampol, 1982). Pericytes have contractile properties and, if damaged, can impair autoregulation, leading to a self-perpetuating cycle of damage to the retinal vasculature (Kuwabara and Cogan, 1963). Hypertension and increased retinal blood flow will also lead to capillary hypertension, since the hydrostatic pressure will be more easily transmitted to the smaller vessels if there is impaired autoregulation. Circumferential stress damage could lead to microaneurysm formation, retinal exudates and oedema, especially as there is no lymphatic drainage of the central nervous system tissues (Milnor, 1989). At the capillary level in diabetes there is increased blood viscosity, decreased red cell deformability and increased platelet aggregation.

The above mentioned changes, along with hyperglycaemia, result in retinal ischaemia, which in turn is a potent stimulus leading to the production of angiogenic and vasoproliferative factors (Patz, 1984). The latter factors lead to new vessel formation and increased retinal blood flow. Increased flow, increased viscosity and capillary closure, all of which occur in diabetes, tend to increase shear stress, resulting in endothelial damage. Pertinent to the diabetic retinal circulation is the observation that an increase in shear stress stimulates mitosis in endothelial cells and increases their turnover (Davies et al., 1986). A similar study showed that increased shear stress can stimulate both the migration and proliferation of endothelial cells (Ando et al., 1987).

Retinal blood flow increases in patients with diabetic retinopathy. Studies using laser Doppler velocimetry and computerized retinal image analysis have shown increased retinal blood flow in diabetic retinopathy. In brief, retinal blood flow is measured by measuring the Doppler shift produced when a low-power helium–neon laser is focused onto moving red blood cells in a retinal blood vessel. Retinal blood flow was reported to be higher by 33 per cent in background, 69 per cent in preproliferative and 50 per cent in proliferative retinopathy compared with non-diabetics (Patel et al., 1992). This was thought to represent failure of autoregulation, even when the systolic and diastolic blood pressure are well within the limits defined for treatment of hypertension in diabetes.

The most important factors that lead to hyperdynamic circulation in the diabetic circulation are hypertension and hyperglycaemia. The effect of hypertension on retinal blood flow was studied in non-diabetic and diabetic patients under conditions of normoglycaemia and hyperglycaemia (Rassam et al., 1995). In non-diabetics, retinal blood flow remained constant when mean arterial pressure (MAP) was increased by 15 per cent and 30 per cent, but there was a 33 per cent increase in retinal blood flow at 40 per cent increase in MAP. In diabetic patients who were normoglycaemic, retinal blood flow remained constant when MAP was increased by up to 30 per cent, but there was a 49 per cent increase in retinal blood flow when MAP was increased by 40 per cent. In contrast, hyperglycaemic diabetic patients showed increased retinal blood flow of 27 per cent, 67 per cent and 102 per cent when MAP was increased by 15 per cent, 30 per cent and 40 per cent respectively. This study illustrates abnormal autoregulation of hypertension in diabetic subjects which was aggravated by hyperglycaemia (Rassam et al., 1995).

The mechanism whereby hyperglycaemia promotes abnormal retinal autoregulation is unclear. Hyperglycaemia leads to increased retinal lactic acid production, which acts as a stimulus to increase retinal blood flow (Keen and Chlouverakis, 1965). Another proposed mechanism is that the excess intracellular glucose shunted through the sorbitol pathway leads to an increase in the cytoplasmic ratio of free NADH to NAD+ (Tilton et al., 1992). This imbalance is also induced by hypoxia and transient ischaemia. This phenomenon has been described as 'hyperglycaemic

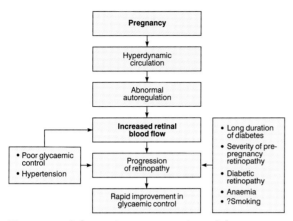

Figure 2.1 Schematic representation of the haemodynamic model incorporating the other known clinical risk factors for the progression of diabetic retinopathy in pregnancy.

pseudohypoxia', and may lead to increased perfusion in the hyperglycaemic state.

Retinal blood flow changes in diabetic pregnancy were studied using the technique of laser Doppler velocimetry (Chen *et al.*, 1994). In diabetic patients, retinal blood flow was found to increase by 14 per cent in the second trimester of pregnancy and by 19 per cent in the third trimester of the pregnancy. There was no significant change in the non-diabetic pregnant control subjects. The diabetes group was then divided into those that had progression of retinopathy and those that remained stable. In the third trimester of pregnancy, retinal blood flow significantly increased by 35 per cent in the diabetic subgroup whose retinopathy deteriorated. In contrast, there was a non-significant increase in retinal blood flow of 5 per cent in the diabetic subgroup that did not have progression of retinopathy. This study shows the haemodynamic model for the pathogenesis of diabetic retinopathy may apply to the progression of retinopathy in pregnancy. A schematic representation of the haemodynamic model incorporating the other known clinical risk factors for the progression of diabetic retinopathy in pregnancy is presented in Figure 2.1. Table 2.1 summarizes the risk factors and their effects.

Conclusion

The study of diabetic retinopathy in pregnancy continues to lead to advancement in our knowledge about the natural history of

Table 2.1 Clinical risk factors in the progression of diabetic retinopathy in pregnancy: effect on retinal blood flow

Factor	Comment	Effect on retinal blood flow
Poor glycaemic control	Aim HBA1c% < 7%	Increase
Rapid improvement in glycaemic control	Aim to improve by no more than 1% HBA1c per month	Decrease, resulting in lesions of retinal ischaemia
Duration of diabetes	Especially duration > 10 years	Probable increase
Hypertension	Aim less than 140/80 mmHg	Increase
	Aim pulse pressure less than 50 mmHg	
Hypercholesterolaemia	Aim less than 5 mmol/l, lower for coronary heart disease (CHD) prevention	Unknown
Smoking	Advise against for CHD risk alone	Decrease? Promote critical ischaemia
Alcohol	Standard advice re. alcohol consumption	No change

Table 2.2 Factors in the progression of diabetic retinopathy in pregnancy

- Lack of preconception care
- Lack of retinal screening
- Duration of diabetes >10 years
- Severity of retinopathy at conception
- Elevated HbA1c%, greater than 7%
- Rapid improvement of poor glycaemic control
- Hypertension greater than 140/80
- Diabetic nephropathy
- Pre-eclampsia
- Smoking

Table 2.3 Screening for diabetic retinopathy in pregnancy

- Screen pre-pregnancy with attention to risk factors (hyperglycaemia, hypertension, hyperlipidaemia)
- Screen at booking, 24 weeks, 32 weeks and pre-delivery
- Type 1 or known Type 2 with dilated pupils
- Undilated pupils usually sufficient in true gestational diabetes
- Refer early, especially maculopathy, preproliferative and proliferative retinopathy

diabetic retinopathy and clinical risk factors in the progression of diabetic retinopathy.

Pregnancy is an important risk factor for the progression of diabetic retinopathy. This risk is increased with several potentially correctable factors (Table 2.2). The general principles of the haemodynamic model for the pathogenesis of diabetic retinopathy presented above are also applicable to other diabetic subgroups. Preconception care should include achieving excellent glycaemic control. It is imperative to ensure that the rate of improvement in glycaemic control is not rapid, both before and particularly during pregnancy. Careful retinal evaluation and appropriate ophthalmological referral and follow-up are essential for pregnant women with diabetes (Table 2.3). Retinal screening should include a minimum of one complete retinal examination every trimester, and within 3 months post-partum.

Understanding the clinical risk factors contributing to the progression of diabetic retinopathy in pregnancy is fundamental to the team management of the pregnant diabetic woman. Most cases of sight-threatening diabetic retinopathy in pregnancy can be avoided by this approach.

Acknowledgements

Dr V. Patel remains indebted to his teacher and mentor Professor Eva Kohner.

References

Ando, J., Nomura, H. and Kamiya, A. (1987). The effect of fluid shear stress on the migration and proliferation of cultured endothelial cells. *Microvasc. Res.*, **33**, 62–70.

Axer-Siegel, R., Hod, M., Fink-Cohen, S. *et al.* (1996). Diabetic retinopathy during pregnancy. *Ophthalmology*, **103(11)**, 1815–19.

Ayed, S., Eddi, A., Daghfous, F. *et al.* (1992). Developmental aspects of diabetic retinopathy during pregnancy (in French). *J. Fr. d'Ophthalmol.*, **15(8–9)**, 474–7.

Briese, V., Straube, W. and Glockner, E. (1991). Serum concentrations of pregnancy-associated alpha-2-glycoprotein in diabetic pregnancy complicated by nonfulminant and proliferative retinopathy. *Zentral. Gynakol.*, **113(19)**, 1042–5.

Brinchmann-Hansen, O., Dahl-Jorgensen, K., Sandvik, L. and Hanssen, K. F. (1992). Blood glucose concentrations and progression of diabetic retinopathy: the seven-year results of the Oslo Study. *Br. Med. J.*, **304**, 19–22.

Chen, H. C., Newsom, R. S. B., Patel, V. *et al.* Retinal blood flow changes during pregnancy in women with diabetes. *Inv. Ophthalmol. Vis. Sci.*, **35(8)**, 3199–208.

Chew, E. Y., Mills, J. L., Metzger, B. E. *et al.* (1995). Metabolic control and progression of retinopathy. The National Institute of Child Health and Human Development Diabetes in Early Pregnancy Study. *Diabetes Care*, **18(5)**, 631–7.

Davies, P. F., Remuzzi, A., Gordon, E. J. *et al.* (1986). Turbulent fluid shear stress induces vascular endothelial cell turnover in vitro. *Proc. Natl. Acad. Sci.* USA, **83**, 2114–17.

DCCT Research Group (1993). The effect of intensive treatment of diabetes on the development and progression of long-term complication in insulin-dependent diabetes mellitus. *N. Engl. J. Med.,* **329**, 977–86.

Garner, A., Ashton, N., Tripathi, R. *et al.* (1975). Pathogenesis of hypertensive retinopathy. An experimental study in the monkey. *Br. J. Ophthalmol.,* **59**, 3–44.

Hagay, Z. J., Schachter, M., Pollack, A. and Levy, R. (1994). Development of proliferative retinopathy in gestational diabetes patient following rapid metabolic control. *Eur. J. Obst. Gyn. Rep. Biol.,* **57(3)**, 211–13.

Hill, D. J., Flyvbjerg, A., Arany, E. *et al.* (1997). Increased levels of serum fibroblast growth factor-2 in diabetic pregnant women with retinopathy. *J. Endocrinol. Metab.,* **82(5)**, 1452–7.

Hopp, H., Vollert, W., Ebert, A. *et al.* (1995). Diabetic retinopathy and nephropathy – complications in pregnancy and labor (in German). *Geburts. Frauenheilkunde,* **55(5)**, 275–9.

Jovanovic-Peterson, L. and Peterson, C. M. (1991). Diabetic retinopathy (review). *Clin. Obst. Gynaecol.,* **34(3)**, 516–25.

Keen, H. and Chlouverakis, C. (1965). Metabolic factors in diabetic retinopathy. In: *Biochemistry of the Retina* (C. N. Graymore, ed.). New York Academic Press.

Klein, B. E., Moss, S. E. and Klein, R. (1990). Effect of pregnancy on progression of diabetic retinopathy. *Diabetes Care,* **13(1)**, 34–40

KROC Collaborative Study Group (1984). Blood glucose control and the evolution of diabetic retinopathy and albuminuria. *N. Engl. J. Med.,* **311**, 365–72.

Kuwabara, T. and Cogan, D. G. (1963). Retinal vascular patterns (VI): mural cells of the retinal capillaries. *Arch. Ophthalmol.,* **69**, 492–502.

Laatikainen, L., Teramo, K., Hieta-Heikurainen, H. *et al.* (1987). A controlled study of the influence of continuous subcutaneous insulin infusion treatment on diabetic retinopathy during pregnancy. *Acta Med. Scand.,* **221(4)**, 367–76.

Milnor, W. R. (1989). *Hemodynamics,* pp. 140–41. Williams & Wilkins.

Moloney, J. B. and Drury, M. I. (1982). The effect of pregnancy on the natural course of diabetic retinopathy. *Am. J. Ophthalmol.,* **93(6)**, 745–56.

Patel, V., Rassam, S., Newsom, R. *et al.* (1992). Retinal blood flow in diabetic retinopathy. *Br. Med. J.,* **305**, 678–83.

Patz, A. (1984). Retinal neovascularization: early contributions of Professor Michaelson and recent observations. *Br. J. Ophthalmol.,* **68**, 42–6.

Phelps, R. L., Sakol, P., Metzger, B. E. *et al.* (1986). Changes in diabetic retinopathy during pregnancy. Correlations with regulation of hyperglycaemia. *Arch. Ophthalmol.,* **104(12)**, 1806–10.

Poulson, J. E. (1953). The Houssay phenomenon in man: recovery from retinopathy in a case of diabetes with Simmond's disease. *Diabetes,* **2**, 7–12.

Rassam, S. M. B., Patel, V. and Kohner, E. M. (1995). The effect of experimental hypertension on retinal vascular autoregulation in humans: a mechanism for the progression of diabetic retinopathy. *Exper. Physiol.,* **80**, 53–68.

Soubrane, G., Canivet, J. and Coscas, G. (1985). Influence of pregnancy on the evolution of background diabetic retinopathy. Preliminary results of a prospective fluorescein angiography study. *Int. Ophthalmol.,* **8(4)**, 249–55.

The Diabetes Control and Complications Trial Research Group (1993). The effect of intensive treatment of diabetes on the development and progression of long-term complications in insulin-dependent diabetes mellitus. *N. Engl. J. Med.,* **329**, 977–86.

Tilton, R. G., Baier, L. D., Harlow, J. E. *et al.* (1992). Diabetes induced glomerular dysfunction: links to a more reduced cytosolic redox ratio of NADH/NAD+. *Kidney Int.,* **41**, 778–88.

Tso, M. O. M. and Jampol, L. M. (1982). Pathophysiology of hypertensive retinopathy. *Ophthalmology,* **89**, 1132–45.

UKPDS Group (1998). Intensive glucose control with sulphonylurea or insulin compared with conventional treatment and risk of complication with type 2 diabetes (UKPDS 33). *Lancet,* **352**, 837–53.

Chapter 3

Histopathology and pathogenesis of diabetic retinopathy

John G. Lawrenson

Introduction

Diabetic retinopathy is a common complication of both Type 1 and Type 2 diabetes mellitus (Klein *et al.*, 1984; Harris *et al.*, 1992), and is the major cause of registerable blindness in the working population in Western countries. As with the equivalent pathological changes in the kidney (nephropathy) and peripheral nervous system (neuropathy), diabetic retinopathy is principally a disorder of small blood vessels (microangiopathy). The Diabetic Control and Complications Trial (DCCT, 1993) provided strong evidence for a causal relationship between hyperglycaemia and diabetic retinopathy; however, despite intensive research the exact mechanism by which raised blood and tissue glucose causes tissue damage is still equivocal (Giardino and Brownlee, 1996). This chapter describes the morphological changes in retinal blood vessels seen in diabetes, and reviews the histopathology of the resulting ophthalmoscopic lesions. Current theories for the pathogenesis of diabetic retinopathy will also be highlighted.

The normal retinal microvasculature

Blood vessels are distributed within the inner two-thirds of the retina, and although their precise arrangement is subject to some regional variability, vessels are typically restricted to particular retinal layers (Figure 3.1). Arterioles and venules are located within the nerve fibre layer, and a rich plexus of capillaries is located at the level of the inner nuclear layer. A capillary-free zone extends around the fovea, whose nutritional requirements are met by the choroid and perifoveal vascular arcades.

Structurally, the wall of a typical retinal capillary is formed by endothelial cells and pericytes surrounded by a basement membrane (Figure 3.2). Endothelial cells are non-fenestrated, and adjacent cells are joined by complex tight junctions (zonula occludens). Pericytes form a discontinuous layer outside the endothelium. A variety of roles have been proposed for these ubiquitous perivascular cells, including mechanical support, local control of blood flow and the control of endothelial cell division (Hirschi and D'Amore, 1996). The vascular basement membrane, which forms a covering around the endothelium and pericyte, is composed predominantly of collagen, glycoproteins and proteoglycans (Ashton, 1974). The basement membrane is an important determinant of vascular permeability, and plays an important role in angiogenesis.

Retinal neurones are very sensitive to changes in their extracellular ion concentration, and many circulating components of the blood are potentially neurotoxic. In order to maintain homeostasis, retinal blood vessels display a selective permeability barrier. The structural basis of this barrier is the tight interendothelial junctions which effectively prevent the paracellular transport of ions and hydrophilic molecules from the bloodstream into the tissue (Cunha-Vaz *et al.*, 1966; Raviola, 1977). An outer permeability barrier, formed by tight

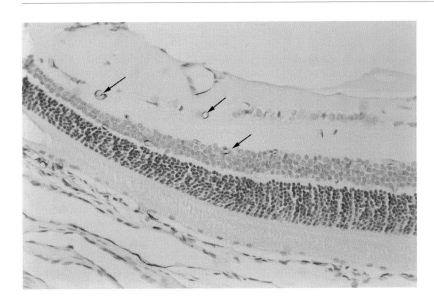

Figure 3.1 Histological section through the retina. An endothelial marker antibody labels retinal microvessels (arrowed). Larger vessels (arterioles and venules) are found within the nerve fibre layer. Only capillaries penetrate to the deeper retinal layers.

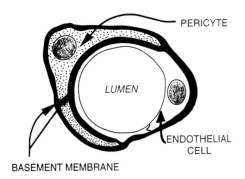

Figure 3.2 Schematic representation of a retinal capillary.

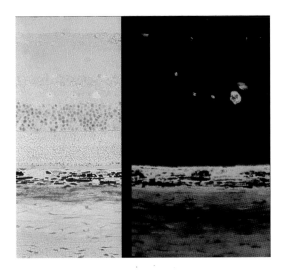

Figure 3.3 Demonstration of the blood–retinal barrier. The micrograph on the right shows a histological section through the retina following an intravenous injection of fluorescein. Note that the fluorescein is confined to the lumen of retinal blood vessels. The retinal pigment epithelium prevents fluorescein leaking into the retina from the choroidal vasculature. The micrograph on the left is included as a reference to location. (Reproduced from Spalton *et al.* (1984) by permission of Mosby.)

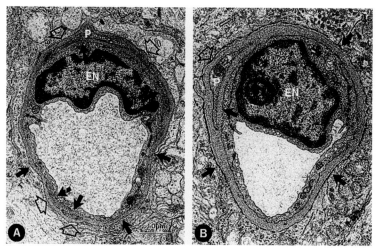

Figure 3.4 (a) Electron micrograph of a normal retinal capillary. Arrows indicate the basement membrane. (b) Retinal capillary from a diabetic retina. Note the thickening of the basement membrane. EN, endothelial cell nucleus; P, pericyte process.

junctions between cells of the retinal pigment epithelium, similarly serves to regulate the free passage of blood-borne solutes from the choroid into the retina. Clinically, the integrity of the blood–retinal barrier is assessed by fluorescein angiography. Following intravenous injection of sodium fluorescein approximately 90 per cent of the fluorescein is bound to serum albumin, and under normal circumstances this fluorescein–protein complex does not cross the vessel wall (Figure 3.3). Manifest fluorescein leakage is evidence of a compromised blood–retinal barrier.

Histopathology of retinal lesions in diabetes retinopathy

Background retinopathy

Subtle histological changes in microvessels are present from earliest stages of this non-proliferative phase of the disease. Microaneurysms are the first ophthalmoscopically visible retinal lesions, followed by intraretinal haemorrhages and hard exudates as the blood–retinal barrier becomes compromised (Dowler and Hamilton, 1996). Mild venous abnormalities and small numbers of cotton wool spots are found in more severe forms of background retinopathy (ETDRS, 1991)

Structural changes in microvessels There are three types of structural change associated with microvessels in diabetes:

- basement membrane thickening
- selective pericyte loss
- endothelial cell damage.

Basement membrane thickening, although not pathognomic for diabetic retinopathy, is an early histological feature of the disease (Ashton, 1974). Measurements of capillary basement membrane thickness in the diabetic retina show a three- to five-fold increase compared to controls (Figure 3.4). The underlying cause of the process is unclear. Possibilities include increased synthesis or reduced degradation, which may be augmented by trapping of plasma proteinaceous material as capillaries become more permeable (Ashton, 1974). Other basement membrane changes seen in diabetes include vacuolization and the presence of lipid inclusions (Ashton, 1974). Associated alterations in its biochemical composition are also likely.

Selective pericyte loss is a unique feature of diabetic microangiopathy, and was first observed in autopsy diabetic retinas. Digestion with the proteolytic enzyme trypsin to remove non-vascular tissue enabled clear visualization

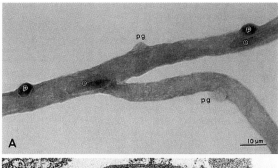

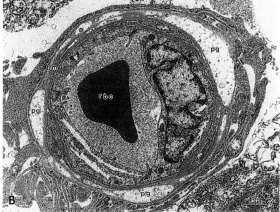

Figure 3.5 (a) Trypsin digest of a diabetic retina showing pericyte ghosts (pg). e, endothelial cell; p, normal pericyte. (b) Electron micrograph of a pericyte ghost showing extensive cytoplasmic degeneration. bm, basement, membrane; rbc, red blood cell.

of the intact retinal vasculature (Cogan *et al.*, 1961). When these trypsin digests are stained and examined microscopically, precise differentiation between endothelial cells and pericytes is possible (Figure 3.5a). In non-diabetic eyes the ratio of pericytes to endothelial cells is approximately 1:1, whereas in diabetics the ratio increases to approximately 1:4, which is suggestive of selective pericyte loss (Cogan and Kuwabara, 1967). Evidence of pericyte degeneration in these digests is provided by the presence of pericyte 'ghosts'. These represent basement membrane pockets marking the space from which the cell contents have disappeared (Figure 3.5a). Electron microscopy confirms the extensive degeneration of the pericyte cytoplasm (Robison *et al.*, 1995; Figure 3.5b).

Endothelial cells play an important role in regulating blood flow by releasing chemical factors that determine the state of contraction of vascular smooth muscle (Grunwald and Bursell, 1996). One early response to hyperglycaemia is changes in retinal blood flow, which in part results from the inability of the endothelial cell to respond to changes in perfusion pressure (autoregulation), producing damaging shear forces. The endothelium is also important for the maintenance of the integrity of the blood–retinal barrier, and endothelial damage in the diabetic retina leads to increased vascular permeability. Later in the course of the disease endothelial cell death occurs, leaving empty tubes of basement membrane (acellular capillaries) which ultimately become non-perfused.

Microaneurysm formation Ophthalmoscopically, microaneurysms appear as dark red spots (10–100 µm in diameter) which show discrete hyperfluorescence on angiography. Trypsin digest preparations of diabetic retina show a

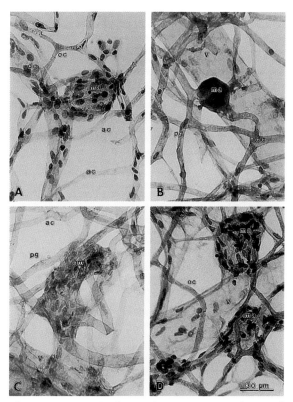

Figure 3.6 Trypsin digest showing various forms of microaneurysm (ma).

variety of morphological forms; divided broadly into cellular and acellular varieties (Figure 3.6; Robison *et al.*, 1995; Stitt *et al.*, 1995). There is general agreement that microaneurysms are strongly associated with pericyte loss, although the precise mechanism involved in their formation is not completely resolved. One view is that they represent focal proliferation of endothelial cells, i.e. an abortive neovascular response (Robison *et al.*, 1995). However, a recent ultrastructural investigation provides evidence for an alternative hypothesis (Stitt *et al.*, 1995). This study suggests that pericyte loss produces a weakening of the endothelial wall and, in conjunction with high capillary perfusion pressure, causes microaneurysm formation. The process starts with focal occlusion by red cells or leukocytes (cellular microaneurysms), which subsequently degenerate and ultimately become completely sclerosed (acellular microaneurysms) (Stitt *et al.*, 1995). The microaneurysm count can be used clinically as a predictor of progression to proliferative diabetic retinopathy (Klein *et al.*, 1989).

Vascular permeability changes: exudates, haemorrhages and oedema Ophthalmoscopic evidence of a compromised blood–retinal barrier is the presence of exudates, haemorrhages and oedema. Hard exudates represent leakage of plasma components, and are yellowish in appearance and often form as a circinate pattern around leaky vessels. Histologically, they consist of aggregates of lipoproteinaceous material and lipid-filled macrophages located at the level of the outer plexiform layer (Figure 3.7; Garner, 1993).

A further disruption of the blood–retinal barrier leads to the passage of the cellular elements of blood across the vessel wall, with the formation of intraretinal haemorrhages. The appearance of the haemorrhage depends on its location within the retina. For example, leakage of blood in the nerve fibre layer produces a superficial 'flame'-shaped haemorrhage as the blood tracks between nerve axons. Haemorrhages in the deeper layers of the retina are of the 'dot and blot' type, which are darker and more circumscribed. Blood is prevented from spreading laterally by Muller cells, which extend vertically through the full thickness of the retina (Garner, 1993).

A breakdown of the blood–retinal barrier in the vicinity of the macula leads to focal or diffuse oedema, which is often associated with haemorrhages and exudates (Dowler and Hamilton, 1996). In severe cases, pooling of extravasated fluid creates cystoid spaces in the inner retinal layers (cystoid macula oedema; Figure 3.8).

Cotton wool spot formation: capillary non-perfusion Capillary non-perfusion is typically

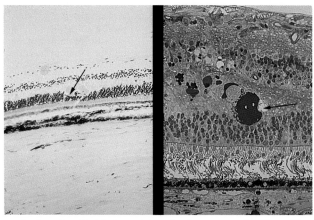

Figure 3.7 Retinal micrograph showing lipid deposition in the outer plexiform layer (arrowed), which is seen clinically as a hard exudate. (Reproduced from Spalton *et al.* (1984) by permission of Mosby.)

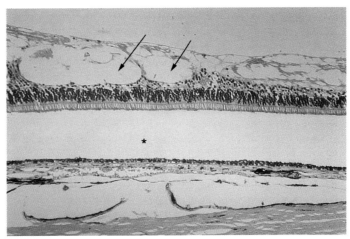

Figure 3.8 Histological section showing cystoid macular oedema. Note the cystoid spaces in the inner retinal layers (arrows). The separation between retina (*) and RPE is an artifact of preparation. (Reproduced from Spalton *et al.* (1984) by permission of Mosby.)

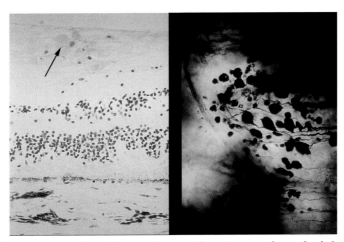

Figure 3.9 Histological appearance of a cotton wool spot. The micrograph on the left shows the position of the lesion in the nerve fibre layer (arrow). The silver stained preparation on the right clearly shows the dilation of nerve axons. (Reproduced from Spalton *et al.* (1984) by permission of Mosby.)

preceded by vascular occlusion. Historically this process has been considered to be due to increased platelet stickiness; however, more recent findings have implicated activated leukocytes in capillary plugging (Schroder *et al.*, 1991). Cotton wool spots occur in association with these discrete areas of non-perfusion. Histologically, they appear as spherical or oval aggregates within the retinal nerve fibre layer (Figure 3.9). Cotton wool spots are sometimes referred to as soft exudates, but this term is a misnomer since they are not formed by an exudative process. Electron microscopic observations indicate that cotton wool spots represent swollen nerve axons of ganglion cells and contain their accumulative debris of degenerated axoplasmic organelles (Figure 3.10). It is thought that the swelling arises from an interruption of axoplasmic transport along the nerve fibre (McLeod *et al.*, 1977). The presence of isolated cotton wool spots has little predictive power for impending neovascularization. However, multiple lesions (more than five) indicates greater capillary

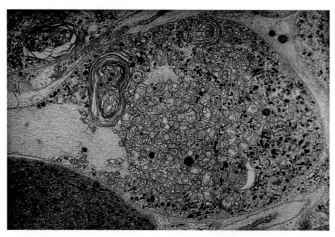

Figure 3.10 Electron micrograph through a cotton wool spot showing a swollen axon containing degenerated axoplasmic organelles. (Reproduced from Spalton *et al.* (1984) by permission of Mosby.)

non-perfusion and significantly increases the risk of progression to the proliferative stage (EDTRS, 1991).

Pre-proliferative retinopathy

Pre-proliferative changes include:

- venous beading
- multiple cotton wool spots (more than five)
- intraretinal microvascular abnormalities
- multiple haemorrhages.

These changes are indicative of severe capillary closure and are associated with a high risk of progression into the proliferative phase of the disease (ETDRS, 1991).

Intraretinal microvascular anbnormalities Intraretinal microvascular abnormalities (IRMA) are defined as retinal vessels showing abnormal branching patterns and irregular focal dilations. They can be differentiated from new vessels since they lie entirely within the retina. Fluorescein angiography indicates that IRMA usually lie at the margins of areas of non-perfusion although, contrary to extraretinal new vessels, they do not leak fluorescein (Dowler and Hamilton, 1996). However, a recent clinicopathological investigation (Imesch *et al.*, 1997) showed that IRMA possess

some morphological features in common with new vessels, i.e. short intercellular junctions and occasional fenestrations. This supports the concept that IRMA have a particular potential for neovascularization.

Proliferative retinopathy

Proliferative retinopathy is characterized by active growth of new vessels which, if untreated, are associated with poor visual prognosis. In advanced retinopathy, severe intraocular ischaemia is associated with neovascularization of the anterior uvea (rubeosis iridis) with the subsequent risk of secondary glaucoma (Dowler and Hamilton, 1996).

Neovascularization and late sequelae of diabetic retinopathy Active new vessel growth, occurring at the disc or elsewhere in the retinal, typically arises from the venous side of the circulation (possibly due to lower oxygen tensions) and progresses through several stages (Figure 3.11) which are under the control of vascular growth factors and other chemical mediators.

Proliferating endothelial cells breach the basement membrane, forming a capillary sprout. The sprout is extended by further endothelial proliferation and is then canalized to forming a capillary tube, which becomes

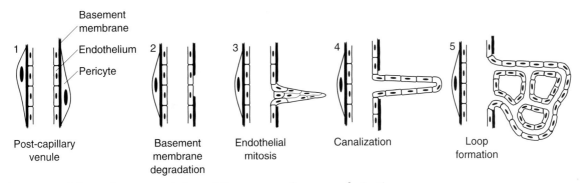

Figure 3.11 Schematic representation of the process of neovascularization.

invested by migrating perivascular cells. The resulting network of new vessels crosses the inner limiting membrane of the retina into the subhyaloid space.

New vessels lack the morphological features of the mature retinal vasculature, i.e. they have reduced numbers of pericytes and display incomplete tight intercellular junctions and occasional fenestrations (Garner, 1993). These features explain why new vessels are prone to leakage and haemorrhage. New vessel formation is associated with the proliferation of fibroblasts and the formation of abnormal attachments to the vitreous gel. As this fibrotic tissue contracts, tractional forces may lead to haemorrhage, retinal tear formation and subsequent detachment (Dowler and Hamilton, 1996).

Pathogenesis of diabetic vascular complications

Using a variety of experimental methods, we have begun to unravel some of the basic biochemical events that are responsible for structural changes in microvessels and new vessel formation. An understanding of these fundamental mechanisms is important, as pharmacological manipulation of these processes is likely to form the basis of future medical therapy for diabetic vascular complications. Animal models have proved useful in the development of knowledge in this area, and can be used to test therapeutic agents (Enger-

man and Kern, 1995). As a model of diabetic retinopathy, the rat offers several practical advantages over larger animals such as dogs and primates. Rat models of both Type 1 and Type 2 diabetes have been developed which show many of the structural changes seen in the human condition (Engerman and Kern, 1995; Robison *et al.*, 1995).

Biochemical pathways underlying the structural changes in microvessels

The clear causal relationship between chronic hyperglycaemia and diabetic microvascular disease (DCCT, 1993) suggests that particular glucose-related metabolic pathways play a role in the vascular pathology seen in diabetes. This is particularly true in tissues like the retina, which do not depend on insulin for glucose uptake. In these insulin-independent tissues, intracellular glucose concentrations rise in parallel with hyperglycaemia (Giardino and Brownlee, 1996). Several metabolic pathways may be involved in glucose mediated tissue damage:

- the polyol pathway
- the diacylglycerol/protein kinase C pathway
- the formation of non-enzymatic glycation products.

The relative importance of each of these pathways is still open to debate but, given the multifactorial nature of the disease, it is likely that each has some responsibility for the pathological changes seen in diabetic micro-angiopathy. Any proposed biochemical mechanism must, however, explain 'hyperglycaemic memory' (Giardino and Brownlee, 1996) – i.e the persistence of glucose-induced microvascular damage once hyperglycaemia has been normalized.

The polyol pathway The polyol pathway converts hexose sugars (e.g. glucose and galactose) into sugar alcohols (polyols). For example, glucose is converted into sorbitol via the action of the enzyme aldose reductase (Figure 3.12). Sorbitol can subsequently be oxidized to fructose, although this conversion occurs very slowly.

Aldose reductase is the rate-limiting enzyme for the pathway. Under normal circumstances aldose reductase has a low affinity for glucose, and in normoglycaemia glucose is principally metabolized by hexokinase (the first enzyme of the glycolytic pathway). However, in hyperglycaemia high intracellular glucose levels saturate hexokinase, and the proportion of glucose converted by the polyol pathway increases. It has been suggested that this increased flux through the polyol pathway plays a significant role in the pathogenesis of diabetic retinopathy (Robison *et al.*, 1995). Enhanced aldose reductase activity and sorbitol accumulation has been reported in the retina of diabetic animals. Since sorbitol does not easily diffuse across cell membranes, it can increase intracellular tonicity and cause cellular damage by an osmotic process. Furthermore, increased polyol pathway activity would alter the redox state of the pyridine nucleotides NADPH and NAD+. Since these are important co-factors in many enzyme-catalysed reactions, other metabolic pathways may be affected. In retinal capillaries the highest level of aldose reductase is found in pericytes (Akagi *et al.*, 1983), and in cell culture experiments pericyte degeneration has been shown to occur in response to accumulated intracellular sorbitol.

Inhibitors of aldose reductase have been synthesized, e.g. sorbinil and tolrestat, and some limited success has been achieved in reducing retinopathy in animal models of diabetes, although a clear beneficial effect has not been seen in human clinical trials (SRTRG, 1990).

The diacylglycerol/protein kinase C pathway The importance of the diacylglycerol/protein kinase C (DAG/PKC) pathway was first demonstrated in cultured vascular cells exposed to high glucose, and later in animal models of diabetes (King, 1996). Diacylglycerol is a phospholipid precursor which is synthesized from intermediates of the glycolytic pathway, glyceraldehyde 3 phosphate and dihydroxyacetone phosphate, or alternatively via the breakdown of phosphatidyl choline. Hyperglycaemia produces corresponding increases in the levels of diacylglycerol, which in turn is linked to the activation of protein kinase C. Functionally, protein kinase C activation affects many vascular properties, including permeability, contractility and basement membrane synthesis. Experimental inhibition of the DAG/PKC pathway can reverse some of the vascular changes seen in the retinas of diabetic animals (King, 1996).

The formation of non-enzymatic glycation products A further consequence of hyperglycaemia is the formation of modified proteins known as glycation products (Brownlee, 1996; Giardino and Brownlee, 1996). These compounds are formed non-enzymatically via a series of intermediate steps (Figure 3.13).

The process is initiated by the attachment of glucose to the amino groups of proteins, forming a Schiff base, which quickly undergoes a chemical modification (Amadori rearrangement) to produce early glycation products. The best known example of such a modified protein is glycosylated haemoglobin (HbA1c), which is monitored clinically as an index of glycaemic control. Early glycation products can combine

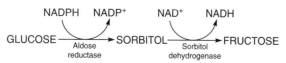

Figure 3.12 The polyol pathoway.

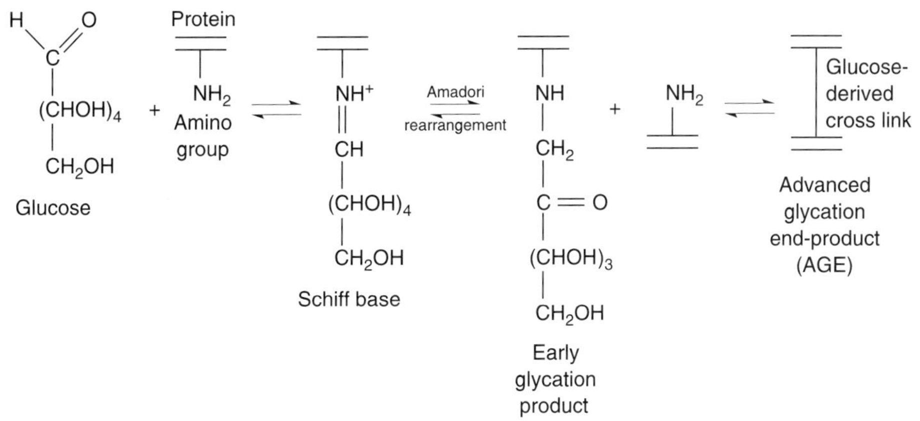

Figure 3.13 Non-enzymatic glycation pathway.

irreversibly with each other to form cross-linked proteins termed advanced glycation end products (AGE). These molecules are stable and long-lived, and therefore do not return to normal once hyperglycaema has been controlled. AGE modification of proteins can occur both intracellularly and extracellularly, leading to an alteration of their functional properties and turnover. Many studies have linked AGE formation to the pathological changes seen in diabetic angiopathy (Giardino and Brownlee, 1996) via several possible mechanisms:

- AGE-modified collagen and laminin (important components of basement membranes) are less susceptible to proteolytic degradation. Accumulation of these abnormal proteins may therefore be responsible for the basement membrane thickening seen in early diabetic retinopathy. Furthermore, glycation of the basement membrane matrix of cultured vascular cells has been shown to affect their proliferation (Kalfa *et al.*, 1995).
- AGE formation within the endothelial cell basement membrane inactivates endothelial-derived nitric oxide, which acts on perivascular smooth muscle causing vasodilation. This may result in impaired blood flow.
- Several cells, including vascular endothelial cells, possess receptors for AGE (Brownlee, 1996). Binding of AGE to the endothelial

receptor causes changes in vascular permeability and favours thrombosis at the endothelial cell surface.

Pharmacological inhibition of AGE formation in experimental diabetes using the drug amino-guanidine offers strong support for the involvement of glycation products in the pathogenesis of diabetic retinopathy. In one study, amino-guanidine treatment resulted in a significant reduction in acellular capillaries and microaneurysms in the diabetic retina (Hammes *et al.*, 1995). Currently, a large, multicentred, randomized trial is underway to look at the effectiveness of the drug in human subjects.

The role of growth factors in ocular neovascularization

In 1948, the British ophthalmologist Isaac Michaelson (Michaelson, 1948) proposed the hypothesis that the stimulus for new vessel growth in vasoproliferative disorders such as diabetic retinopathy arose from the retina itself. This notion was extended by the work of Ashton (Ashton, 1949; Ashton, 1963) and others who observed that neovascularization was always preceded by capillary non-perfusion, thereby establishing a link between ischaemia and the signal for new vessel growth. The identity of the putative angiogenesis factor has been a mystery for almost half a century.

The principal difficulty was the diverse range of attributes that such a molecule must possess in order to account for the observed pathology, i.e.

- it must stimulate angiogenesis
- it must be produced in response to low oxygen levels
- it should be consistently found in eyes with proliferative retinopathy
- it should be diffusible, in order to account for vascularization at sites distant from the retina, e.g. rubeosis iridis
- its level should decrease following any treatment that reduces neovascularization.

Although several growth factors have been proposed to play a role in proliferative diabetic retinopathy, e.g. basic fibroblast growth factor (bFGF) and insulin-like growth factor (IGF), until recently no one molecule has been able to fulfil all of the above criteria. However, developments over the last few years have identified an angiogenesis factor that offers considerable promise (Aiello, 1997). Vascular endothelial growth factor (VEGF) was first discovered in the 1980s as a molecule which attracted blood vessels to tumours, although at that time it was principally noted for its effect on vascular permeability (50 000 times more potent than histamine) (Senger et al., 1990). It was not until it was demonstrated that VEGF production was linked to hypoxia (Shweiki et al., 1992) that it became a candidate for the angiogenesis signal in proliferative retinopathies.

Working initially with cultured vascular cells, and later in animal models of neovascularization, researchers have demonstrated a clear temporal and spatial relationship between VEGF production and new vessel growth (Aiello, 1997). Furthermore, several studies have identified VEGF expression in human eyes with proliferative diabetic retinopathy (Adamis et al., 1994; Aiello et al., 1994; Malecaze et al., 1994). Because VEGF also has vasopermeability properties, it may additionally mediate the hyperpermeability observed in diabetic retinopathy.

The identification of VEGF as a major factor in the pathogenesis of neovascularization has considerable therepeutic implications. Currently, treatment options in proliferative retinopathy are limited. Panretinal photocoagulation is effective although, by destroying large areas of peripheral retina, the treatment is associated with significant side effects.

VEGF inhibition studies in experimental animals have been evaluated, and early results are very promising (Aiello et al., 1995; Robinson et al., 1996). However, drug delivery and safety issues still need to be addressed before clinical trials of VEGF inhibitors can be undertaken.

References

Adamis, A. P., Miller, J. W., Bernal, M. T. et al. (1994). Increased vascular endothelial growth factor levels in the vitreous of eyes with proliferative diabetic retinopathy. Am. J. Ophthalmol., **118**, 445–50.

Aiello, L. P. (1997). Clinical implications of vascular growth factors in proliferative retinopathies. Curr. Opin. Ophthalmol., **8**, 19–31.

Aiello, L. P., Avery, R. L., Arrig, P. G. et al. (1994). Vascular endothelial growth factor in ocular fluid of patients with diabetic retinopathy and other retinal disorders. N. Engl. J. Med., **331**, 1480–87.

Aiello, L. P., Pierce, E. A., Foely, E. D. et al. (1995). Inhibition of vascular endothelial growth factor supresses reteinal neovascularization in vivo. Proc. Natl. Acad. Sci. USA, **92**, 10457–61.

Akagi, Y., Kador, P. F., Kuwabara, T. and Kinoshita, J. H. (1983). Aldose reductase localisation in human mural cells. Invest. Ophthalmol. Vis. Sci., **24**, 1516–19.

Ashton, N. (1949). Vascular changes in diabetes with particular reference to the retinal vessels. Preliminary report. Br. J. Ophthalmol., **33**, 407–20.

Ashton, N. (1963). Studies of the retinal capillaries in relation to diabetes and other retinopathies. Br. J. Ophthalmol., **47**, 521–38.

Ashton, N. (1974). Vascular basement membrane changes in diabetic retinopathy. Br. J. Ophthalmol., **58**, 344–66.

Brownlee, M. (1996). Advanced glycation end products in diabetic complications. Curr. Opin. Endocrinol., **3**, 291–7.

Cogan, D. G. and Kuwabara, T. (1967). The mural cell in perspective. Arch. Ophthalmol., **78**, 133–9.

Cogan, D. G., Toussaint, D. and Kuwabara, T. (1961). Retinal vascular patterns IV, diabetic retinopathy. Arch. Ophthalmol., **66**, 366–78.

Cunha-Vaz, J. G., Shakib, M. and Ashton, N. (1966). Studies on the permeability of the blood–retinal barrier I. On the existence, development and site of a blood–retinal barrier. *Br. J. Ophthalmol.*, **50**, 441–53.

Diabetes Control and Complications Trial Research Group (1993). The effect of intensive treatment of diabetes on the development and pathogenesis of long-term complications in insulin-dependent diabetes. *N. Engl. J. Med.*, **329**, 977–86.

Dowler, J. G. F. and Hamilton, A. M. P. (1996). Clinical features of diabetic eye disease. In: *Textbook of Diabetes* (J. C. Pickup and G. Williams, eds). Blackwell Science, 46.1–46.14.

Early Treatment Diabetic Retinopathy Study Research Group (1991). Fundus photographic risk factors for progression of diabetic retinopathy. Study Report 12. *Ophthalmology*, **98**, 823–33.

Engerman, R. L. and Kern, T. S. (1995). Retinopathy in animal models of diabetes. *Diabetes/Met. Rev.*, **11**, 109–20.

Garner, A. (1993). Histopathology of diabetic retinopathy. *Eye*, **7**, 250–53.

Giardino, I. and Brownlee, M. (1996). The biochemical basis of microvascular disease. In: *Textbook of Diabetes* (J. C. Pickup and G. Williams, eds). Blackwell Science, 42.1–42.16.

Grunwald, J. E. and Bursell, S. E. (1996). Hemodynamic changes as early markers of diabetic retinopathy. *Curr. Opin. Endocrinol. Diabetes*, **3**, 298–306.

Hammes, H. P., Strodler, D., Weiss, A. *et al.* (1995) Secondary intervention with aminoguanidine retards the progression of diabetic retinopathy in the rat model. *Diabetologia*, **38**, 656–60.

Harris, M. I., Klein, R., Welborn, T. A. *et al.* (1992). Onset of NIDDM occurs at least 4–7 years before clinical diagnosis. *Diabetes Care*, **15**, 815–19.

Hirschi, K. K. and D'Amore, P. A. (1996). Pericytes in the microvasculature. *Cardiovasc. Res.*, **32**, 687–98.

Imesch, P. D., Bindley, C. D. and Wallow, I. H. (1997). Clinicopathological correlation of intraretinal microvascular abnormalities. *Retina*, **17**, 321–9.

Kalfa, T. A., Gerritsen, M. E., Carlson, E. C. *et al.* (1995). Altered proliferation of retinal vascular cells on a glycated matrix. *Inv. Ophthalmol. Vis. Sci.*, **36**, 2358–67.

King, G. L. (1996) The role of protein kinase C activation in the development of vascular disease in diabetes. *Curr. Opin. Endocrinol.*, **3**, 285–90.

Klein, R., Klein, B. E. K., Moss, S. E. *et al.* (1984). The Winsconsin epidemiological study of diabetic retinopathy. II. Prevalence and risk of diabetic retinopathy when age at diagnosis is less than 30 years. *Arch. Ophthalmol.*, **102**, 520–26.

Klein, R., Meuer, S. M., Moss, S. E. *et al.* (1989). The relationship between retinal microaneurysm counts to the 4-year progression of diabetic retinopathy. *Arch. Ophthalmol.*, **107**, 1780–85.

Malecaze, F., Clamens, S., Simorre-Pinatel, V. *et al.* (1994). Detection of vascular endothelial growth factor messenger RNA and vascular endothelial-like activity in proliferative diabetic retinopathy. *Arch. Ophthalmol.*, **112**, 1476–82.

McLeod, D., Marshall, J., Kohner, E. M. and Bird, A. C. (1977). The role of axoplasmic transport in the pathogenesis of retinal cotton wool spots. *Br. J. Ophthalmol.*, **61**, 177–91.

Michaelson, I. C. (1948). The mode of development of the vascular system of the retina with some observations on its significance for certain retinal diseases. *Trans. Ophthalmol. Soc. UK*, **68**, 137–80.

Raviola, G. (1977). The structural basis of the blood–ocular barriers. *Exp. Eye Res.*, **25** (Suppl), 27–63.

Robinson, G. S., Pierce, E. A., Rook, S. L. *et al.* (1996). Oligodeoxynucleotides inhibit retinal neovascularisation in a murine model of proliferative retinopathy. *Proc. Natl. Acad. Sci. USA*, **93**, 4851–6.

Robison, W. G., Laver, N. M. and Lou, M. F. (1995). The role of aldose reductase in diabetic retinopathy: prevention and intervention studies. *Prog. Retinal Eye Res.*, **14**, 593–641.

Schroder, S., Palinski, W. and Schmid-Schobein, G. W. (1991). Activated monocytes and granulocytes, capillary non-perfusion and neovascularization in diabetic retinopathy. *Am. J. Pathol.*, **139**, 81–100.

Sorbitol Retinopathy Trial Research Group (1990). A randomised trial of sorbinil, an aldose reductase inhibitor, in diabetic retinopathy. *Acta Ophthalmol.*, **108**, 1234–44.

Senger, D., Connolly, D., Van De Water, L. *et al.* (1990). Purification and NH$_2$-terminal amino acid sequence of guinea pig tumor secreted vascular permeability factor. *Cancer Res.*, **50**, 1774–8.

Shweiki, D., Itin, A., Soffer, D., and Keshet, E. (1992). Vascular endothelial growth factor induced by hypoxia may mediate hypoxia-initiated angiogenesis. *Nature*, **359**, 843–5.

Stitt, A. W., Gardiner, T. A. and Archer, D. B. (1995). Histological and ultrastructural investigation of retinal microaneurysm development in diabetic patients. *Br. J. Ophthalmol.*, **79**, 362–7.

Chapter 4

Epidemiology of diabetic eye disease
Gillian C. Vafidis

Introduction

Diabetic eye disease is an important cause of world blindness (Ghafour *et al.*, 1983; National Society to Prevent Blindness, 1993). The study of its epidemiology improves our understanding of diabetic eye disease and suggests ways in which visual loss may be prevented.

The first report of retinal problems in diabetes was by Von Jaeger in Vienna in 1856. Since that time there have been a number of epidemiological studies concerned with diabetic-related eye problems (Stolk *et al.*, 1995; Framingham Eye Study, 1980; Houston, 1982; Foulds *et al.*, 1983), the most comprehensive being The Wisconsin Epidemiologic Study of Diabetic Retinopathy (WESDR), which has reported on over 2300 diabetic inhabitants of Southern Wisconsin, United States (USA) over the last 14 years (Klein *et al.*, 1984a). The findings of this study provide much of the statistical data discussed in this chapter. Table 4.1 defines the epidemiological terms used.

Table 4.1 Definition of epidemiological terms

Term	Definition
Epidemiology	The study of patterns of diseases within populations
Prevalence	The number of cases in a given population at a single point in time
Incidence	The number of new cases in a specified population over a specified time period
Type 1 diabetes	Diabetes diagnosed before the age of 30 years, controlled by insulin injections
Type 2 diabetes	Diabetes diagnosed at or after the age of 30 years, controlled by insulin injection, hypoglycaemic medication or diet alone
Risk factors	Factors that increase the chances of an individual or population developing a specified disease or complication
Relative risk	An assessment of the influence of a risk factor on the rate (or risk) of an event occurring. It measures the strength of an association between a risk factor and disease, but cannot prove a causal relationship between the risk factor and disease
Odds ratio	An approximation to relative risk. It compares the risk of disease in someone with a given risk factor to that in someone without

Epidemiology of blindness in diabetes

Diabetes is the leading cause of blindness in the working population in developed countries. It accounts for 7–8 per cent of all blind registrations and for 1000 new blindness registrations in the UK each year (Evans, 1995), most of which are for diabetic retinopathy. It is the single most important cause of preventable blindness, and it has been estimated that individuals with diabetes have a 25 times higher risk of going blind than those without the disease (Kahn and Hiller, 1974).

Diabetic retinopathy causes blindness in one of two ways, either by direct involvement of the macular capillaries or from the complications of proliferative disease. In young patients, where diabetes is diagnosed before the age of 30 years (Type 1 diabetes), blindness is usually as a consequence of proliferative disease. In people diagnosed after the age of 30 years (Type 2 disease), visual impairment is most frequently due to cataract and blindness from diabetic macular oedema (Klein *et al.*, 1984b). Type 2 disease is associated with the highest incidence of blindness, with 4 per cent of those using insulin and 4.8 per cent of those not using insulin going blind over a 10-year period (Klein *et al.*, 1994a).

Cataract is the major cause of blindness in the developing world (Wilson, 1980). Where malnutrition is common diabetes is uncommon, but as life expectancy and standards of living rise it is anticipated that diabetes and consequently diabetic retinopathy will become a major cause of blindness in the developing world.

Prevalence of diabetic eye disease

Diabetes is estimated to affect 100 million people world-wide. In western countries the prevalence is between 2 and 4 per cent of the population. The majority have 'maturity onset' Type 2 disease, and only 10–15 per cent have Type 1 diabetes, i.e. they developed the disease in childhood or in young adult life. The age at onset determines the frequency and nature of diabetic eye complications.

The major ocular complication of diabetes is retinopathy, which is present in one-third of all individuals with diabetes. Younger onset patients have the highest prevalence and the most severe retinopathy. Less frequent and less severe diabetic retinopathy is found in older onset patients not using insulin (Kahn and Hiller, 1974).

The ocular consequences of diabetes are not confined to retinopathy, and include cataract and cranial nerve palsies. Significant cataract was found in 60 per cent of the diabetic population aged 30–54 years in the WESDR (Klein *et al.*, 1985), a five-fold increased prevalence over that of a control population. Intraocular inflammation, glaucoma and retinal vascular disease are also more commonly found in diabetic patients than in a non-diabetic population.

Diabetic retinopathy

Prevalence of diabetic retinopathy

Diabetic retinopathy principally affects small retinal blood vessels. Its onset and development are related to a number of factors: the type and control of diabetes, concurrent circulatory, hormonal and metabolic problems, and the race, age, sex and diet of the individual.

For both Type 1 and Type 2 diabetes, a consistent predictor of the presence of retinopathy is the duration of the systemic disease. The longer an individual has had diabetes, the more likely is diabetic retinopathy. After 5 years of diabetes, the overall prevalence of any retinopathy is 25 per cent. After 10 years this figure has risen to 60 per cent, and by 15 years 80 per cent of all diabetic individuals will have retinopathy. Type 1 patients demonstrate the strongest relationship between diabetic retinopathy and duration of disease (Palmberg *et al.*, 1981). At diagnosis of Type 1 disease retinopathy is unusual, but by 15 years of diabetes, it is an almost universal finding. A similar association with disease duration occurs in Type 2 diabetes, although significant retinopathy is already present at diagnosis in up to 30 per cent

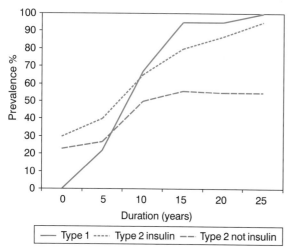

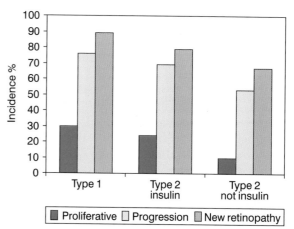

Figure 4.1 Prevalence of diabetic retinopathy with type and duration of disease. The frequency of retinopathy at diagnosis is higher in Type 2 disease. The frequency of retinopathy in Type 1 disease is almost 100 per cent after 15 years' duration. Data from WESDR (Klein *et al.*, 1984a, 1984c).

Figure 4.2 Ten-year incidence and progression of retinopathy with type of diabetes. The incidence of new retinopathy, the progression of existing retinopathy and the incidence of proliferative retinopathy are higher in patients using insulin. Data from WESDR (Klein *et al.*, 1994).

and the frequency of retinopathy never reaches the high prevalence levels of Type 1 disease, even after 25 years (Klein *et al.*, 1984c) (Figure 4.1)

Incidence of retinopathy

The incidence of retinopathy is an index of the development of new or progressive retinal disease occurring within a diabetic population in a specified period of time. Incidence data are especially useful for planning health resources. It is important to be able to estimate the number of people within a population who are likely to develop sight-threatening disease over a given time interval so that appropriate health provision can be planned.

The Wisconsin Study looked at the number of new cases of retinopathy in the study population, and also at progression of retinopathy in those with pathology at the start of the study. When comparing Type 1 with Type 2 diabetes, they found that the highest incidence of new retinopathy was in Type 1 patients. Nearly 60 per cent of Type 1 patients without

retinopathy at the start developed it over a 4-year period. Significant progression of retinopathy also occurred in this group. One in ten of those with non-proliferative disease progressed to proliferative retinopathy within 4 years (Klein *et al.*, 1989a).

In people with Type 2 disease using insulin who did not have any retinopathy at the start of the study, nearly 50 per cent developed new retinopathy and 7 per cent developed proliferative disease after 4 years. Even in Type 2 diabetes controlled on hypoglycaemic medication and/or diet, a third developed new retinopathy and a quarter had progression of existing retinopathy (Klein *et al.*, 1989b). The 10-year incidence and progression of retinopathy is shown in Figure 4.2.

Risk factors

In a given individual, the risk of diabetes is a function of genetic inheritance, age, obesity, level of physical activity, cigarette smoking and alcohol use. Risk factors for diabetic retinopathy have also been identified. These factors

Table 4.2 Known risk factors for the development and progression of diabetic retinopathy

Type 1 (age at onset less than 30 years)	Type 2 (age at onset over 30 years)
Higher blood sugar levels	Higher blood sugar levels
Higher diastolic blood pressure	Higher systolic blood pressure
Gross proteinuria	Presence of proteinuria
Increased age	Use of insulin
Male sex	

influence the type and progression of disease, and offer the hope that by their manipulation the onset of retinopathy may be delayed or prevented altogether.

Genetic risk factors Genetic risk factors are important in both Type 1 and Type 2 diabetes. Specific chromosomal patterns appear to correspond to the development of diabetic retinopathy in Type 1 diabetes. For example, the presence of HLA-B15 histocompatibility antigen increases four-fold the risk of developing retinopathy. Identical twin studies in Type 2 diabetes have shown that equivalent grades of retinopathy in sibling pairs occur significantly more often than can be attributed to chance alone (Barnett *et al.*, 1981).

Blood sugar control Metabolic risk factors are highly significant in the development and progression of diabetic retinopathy. Table 4.2 lists the risk factors for the development and progression of retinopathy. Uncontrolled blood sugar is the most important determinant of the development and progression of diabetic retinopathy so far identified. A large trial in the USA, the Diabetes Control and Complications Trial (DCCT, 1993), found that strict control of blood sugar in Type 1 diabetes reduced the 5-year risk of new retinopathy by 76 per cent and the risk of progression of existing retinopathy by 54 per cent. In Type 2 disease, uncontrolled hyperglycaemia is also recognized to be a risk factor for retinopathy. Data from the WESDR shows the association of 10-year incidence of retinopathy with blood sugar control

at baseline for both Type 1 and Type 2 patients (Klein *et al.*, 1988; Figure 4.3a). In both types of diabetes the incidence of retinopathy is higher if blood sugar is poorly controlled, and progression of retinopathy is also more common in those with worse control (Figure 4.3b). The incidence of proliferative disease and macular oedema are significantly reduced in those with blood sugar levels that are nearer normal levels (Figures 4.3c, 4.3d). These data suggest that better control of blood sugar would lead to a reduction in the incidence of blindness due to diabetes.

Unfortunately, once diabetic retinopathy is well established, better control of blood sugar does not appear to slow progression of the disease (DCCT, 1993), and it is important that near normoglycaemia is established and maintained from diagnosis to prevent blindness in later life.

Use of insulin Insulin use is associated with a higher prevalence of retinopathy (Dwyer *et al.*, 1985). All Type 1 and some Type 2 diabetic individuals need insulin to control their blood sugar. It has been found that those using insulin develop more retinopathy than those using hypoglycaemic medication and diet alone. Both proliferative retinopathy (Palmberg *et al.*, 1981; Klein *et al.*, 1984c; Klein *et al.*, 1989a) and macular oedema (Klein *et al.*, 1984d) are more prevalent in those using insulin. (Figures 4.4, 4.5). Insulin use also influences the incidence of retinopathy. Over a 10-year period, retinopathy developed in more WESDR diabetic patients using insulin than in those

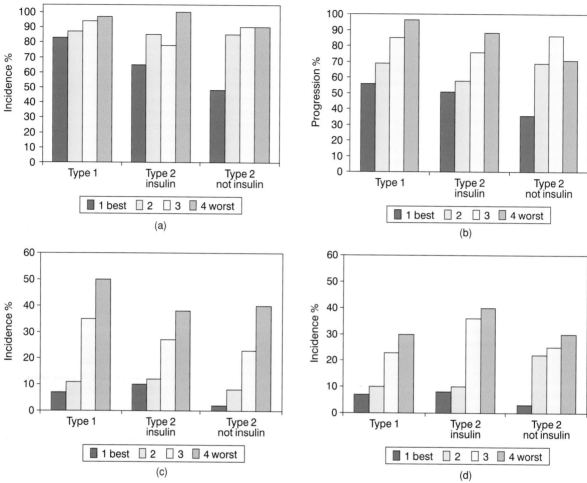

Figure 4.3 (a) Ten-year incidence of new retinopathy by quartiles of blood sugar levels at baseline. In all groups, the best blood sugar control is associated with the least retinopathy. (b) Ten-year progression of retinopathy by quartiles of blood sugar levels at baseline. Better blood sugar levels were associated with less progression of retinopathy. (c) Ten-year incidence of proliferative retinopathy by quartiles of blood sugar levels at baseline. Proliferative disease is significantly less with lower blood sugar levels. (d) Ten-year incidence of macular oedema by quartiles of blood sugar control at baseline. In all cases quartile 1 is the group with lowest blood sugar levels (best control), quartile 2 is the next level up, quartile 3 is higher still and quartile 4 is the group with the the highest blood sugar levels. All data from WESDR (Klein *et al.*, 1988).

controlled by other means (Klein *et al.*, 1994b). Proliferative retinopathy was also more common in patients using insulin (Figure 4.6).

Other risk factors

1. Age is important to the prevalence of retinopathy. Any retinopathy is rare before puberty (Krolewski *et al.*, 1986). Older age is positively related to the presence of diabetic macular oedema in Type 1 and Type 2 diabetes (Klein *et al.*, 1984d). Older age is also a recognized risk factor for severity of retinopathy in Type 1 patients (Moss *et al.*, 1998).

2. Hypertension is an independent risk factor for diabetic retinopathy (UK Prospective Diabetes Study Group, 1998) and visual loss

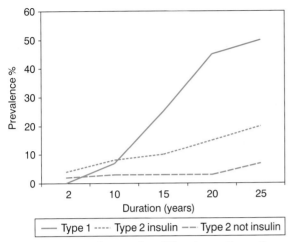

Figure 4.4 Prevalence of proliferative retinopathy by type and control of diabetes. Data from WESDR (Klein *et al.*, 1984a, 1984c).

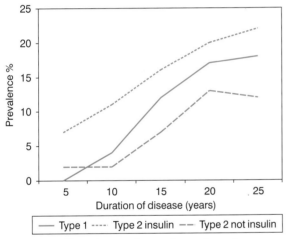

Figure 4.5 Prevalence of macular oedema by duration of disease. Type 2 patients on insulin have the highest prevalence of macular oedema. Data from WESDR (Klein *et al.*, 1984d).

(Sjolie *et al.*, 1997). Abnormally high lipid levels in blood are associated with more retinal exudates (Chew *et al.*, 1996) and progression of retinopathy (Dornan *et al.*, 1982).

3. High alcohol intake is associated with a three-fold increased risk of more severe retinal disease (Moss *et al.*, 1994).

4. Renal disease is also associated with the development and progression of retinopathy (Klein *et al.*, 1993).

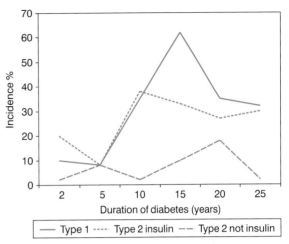

Figure 4.6 Ten-year incidence of proliferative retinopathy by duration of diabetes. Type 2 patients not using insulin have less risk of proliferative retinopathy developing, even after many years of diabetes. Data from WESDR (Klein *et al.*, 1994).

5. Hormonal factors are important. The onset of puberty (Krolewski *et al.*, 1986) and the pregnant state (Sunness, 1988) can result in progression of retinopathy.

In the future, a better understanding of the risk factors will allow construction of a risk profile for each individual patient with regard to the various complications of diabetes. It would then be possible to discuss the risk to sight and how individuals might alter their lifestyle to reduce the development of complications. Fear of blindness may be the incentive needed to improve compliance with diet and good blood sugar control.

More retinopathy in the future?

The reported prevalence of diabetes is rising (O'Rahilly, 1997). In part this may be due to an increasing incidence of diabetes. There is also earlier detection of the disease with longer survival. In part it is because the number of elderly in the population is rising, and diabetes is more prevalent in the elderly.

There is evidence that many of those with retinopathy are being referred too late for effective treatment to prevent visual loss (Jones *et al.*, 1988). In the future, with increasing numbers of diabetic people in society, screening and treatment strategies will need to improve if an associated rise in diabetes-related blindness is to be prevented.

Possible remedies

In recent years there have been a number of important developments in the understanding of the influence of metabolic factors on the progression of diabetic retinopathy. It is now recognized that diabetic retinopathy can be prevented by adherence to a regime which includes strict blood glucose control, low fat diet, regular exercise and avoidance of obesity. There may be other as yet unrecognized risk factors. The challenge is to motivate and educate those with diabetes, especially those who are without complications, so that retinopathy and other diabetic problems can be avoided.

Prevention of blindness

In 1989, representatives from all European countries met to discuss diabetes care. They formulated The St Vincent Declaration, which outlined 5-year targets to reduce the morbidity and mortality from diabetes (The St Vincent Group, 1990). Data from epidemiological studies suggest two public health approaches to achieving these goals; better blood sugar control and better detection and treatment of diabetic retinopathy. The immediate introduction of universal systematic screening of diabetic individuals could achieve the St Vincent goal in the UK, since it is estimated that 60 per cent of diabetes-related blindness is preventable. Sight-threatening disease is often asymptomatic (Klein *et al.*, 1986), and treatment is even more effective if it is carried out before advanced retinopathy develops (The Diabetic Retinopathy Study Research Group, 1979).

To comply with the St Vincent declaration, the UK should introduce immediate regular fundus screening of all diabetic people. Initially, additional treatment facilities would need to be made available to catch up the existing backlog of untreated retinopathy. As measures to achieve better control of blood sugar reduce the incidence of retinal complications, fewer treatment centres would be required. Within two generations, the goal of eliminating the greater part of blindness due to diabetes could be achieved.

References

Barnett, A. H., Eff, C., Leslie, R. D. G. and Pyke, D. A. (1981). Diabetes in identical twins: a study of 200 pairs. *Diabetologia*, **20**, 87–93.

Chew, E. Y., Klein, M. L., Ferris, F. L. *et al.* (1996). Association of elevated serum lipid levels with retinal hard exudate in diabetic retinopathy. ETDRS Report Number 22. *Arch. Ophthalmol.*, **114**, 1079–84.

Evans, J. (1995). *Causes of Blindness and Partial Sight in England and Wales 1990/91*. Studies on Medical and Population Subjects No. 57. HMSO.

Diabetes Control and Complications Trial Research Group (1993). The effect of intensive treatment of diabetes on the development and progression of long-term complications in insulin dependent diabetes mellitus. *New Engl. J. Med.*, **329**, 977–86.

Dornan, T. L., Carter, R. D., Bron, A. J. *et al.* (1982). Low density lipoprotein cholesterol: an association with the severity of diabetic retinopathy. *Diabetologia*, **22**, 167–70.

Dwyer, M. S., Melton, I. J., Ballard, D. J. *et al.* (1985). Incidence of diabetic retinopathy and blindness: a population based study in Rochester, Minnesota. *Diabetes Care*, **8**, 316–22.

Foulds, W. S., McCuish, A., Barrie, T. *et al.* (1983). Diabetic retinopathy in the West of Scotland: Its detection and prevalence and cost-effectiveness of a proposed screening programme. *Health Bull.*, **41**, 318–26.

Framingham Eye Study Monograph (1980). *Surv. Ophthalmol.*, **24**, 401–27.

Ghafour, I. M., Allan, D. and Foulds, W. S. (1983). Common causes of blindness and visual handicap in the West of Scotland. *Br. J. Ophthalmol.*, **67**, 209–13.

Houston, A. (1982). Retinopathy in the Poole area: an epidemiological enquiry. In: *Advances in Diabetes Epidemiology* (E. Eschwege, ed.), pp. 199–206. Elsevier Biomedical Press B.V.

Jones, D., Dolben, J., Owens, D. R. *et al.* (1988). Non-mydriatic polaroid photography in screening for diabetic retinopathy: evaluation in a clinical setting. *Br. Med. J.*, **296**, 1029–30.

Kahn, H. A. and Hiller, R. (1974). Blindness caused by diabetic retinopathy. *Am. J. Ophthalmol.*, **78**, 58–67.

Klein, R., Klein, B. E. K. and Moss, S. E. (1984a). The Wisconsin epidemiologic study of diabetic retinopathy. II. Prevalence and risk of diabetic retinopathy when age at diagnosis is less than 30 years. *Arch. Ophthalmol.*, **102**, 520–26.

Klein, R., Klein, B. E. K. and Moss, S. E. (1984b). Visual impairment in diabetes. *Ophthalmology*, **91**, 1–9.

Klein, R., Klein, B. E. K., Moss, S. E. *et al.* (1984c). The Wisconsin epidemiologic study of diabetic retinopathy. III. Prevalence and risk of diabetic retinopathy when age at diagnosis is 30 or more years. *Arch. Ophthalmol.*, **102**, 527–32.

Klein, R., Klein, B. E. K., Moss, S. E. *et al.* (1984d). The Wisconsin Epidemiologic Study of Diabetic Retinopathy. Diabetic macular oedema. *Ophthalmology*, **91**, 1464–74.

Klein, B. E. K., Klein, R. and Moss, S. E. (1985). Prevalence of cataracts in a population based study of persons with diabetes mellitus. *Ophthalmology*, **92**, 1191–6.

Klein, R., Klein, B. E. K., Moss, S. E. *et al.* (1986). The validity of a survey question to study diabetic retinopathy. *Am. J. Epidemiol.*, **124**, 104–10.

Klein, R., Klein, B. E. K., Moss, S. E. *et al.* (1988). Glycosylated haemoglobin predicts the incidence and progression of diabetic retinopathy. *JAMA*, **260**, 2864–71.

Klein, R., Klein, B. E. K., Moss, S. E. *et al.* (1989a). The Wisconsin epidemiologic study of diabetic retinopathy. IX. Four-year incidence and progression of diabetic retinopathy when age at diagnosis is less than 30 years. *Arch. Ophthalmol.*, **107**, 237–43.

Klein, R., Klein, B. E. K., Moss, S. E. *et al.* (1989b). The Wisconsin epidemiologic study of diabetic retinopathy. X. Four year incidence and progression of diabetic retinopathy when age at diagnosis is 30 years or more. *Arch. Ophthalmol.*, **107**, 244–9.

Klein, R., Moss, S. E. and Klein, B. E. K. (1993). Is gross proteinuria a risk factor for the incidence of proliferative diabetic retinopathy? *Ophthalmology*, **100**, 1140–46.

Klein, R., Klein, B. E. K. and Moss, S. E. (1994a). Ten-year incidence of visual loss in a diabetic population. *Ophthalmology*, **101**, 1061–70.

Klein, R., Klein, B. E. K., Moss, S. E. and Cruickshanks, K. J. (1994b). The Wisconsin Epidemiologic Study of Diabetic Retinopathy. XIV. Ten-year incidence and progression of diabetic retinopathy. *Arch. Ophthalmol.*, **112**, 1217–28.

Krolewski, A. S., Warram, J. H., Rand, L. I. *et al.* (1986). Risk of proliferative diabetic retinopathy in juvenile-onset Type 1 diabetes: a 40-year follow-up study. *Diabetes Care*, **9**, 443–52.

Moss, S. E., Klein, R. and Klein, B. E. K. (1994). The association of alcohol consumption with the incidence and progression of diabetic retinopathy. *Ophthalmology*, **101**, 1962–8.

Moss, S. E., Klein, R. and Klein, B. E. K. (1998). The 14-year incidence of visual loss in a diabetic population. *Ophthalmology*, **105**, 998–1003.

National Society to Prevent Blindness (1993). Vision problems in the US: facts and figures. The American Academy of Ophthalmology Preferred Practice Patterns Series: *Diabetic Retinopathy*, 19–20.

O'Rahilly, S. (1997). Non-insulin dependent diabetes mellitus: The gathering storm. *Br. Med. J.*, **314**, 955–9.

Palmberg, P., Smith, M., Waltman, S. *et al.* (1981). The natural history of retinopathy in insulin dependent juvenile-onset diabetes. *Ophthalmology*, **88**, 613–18.

Sjolie, A. K., Stephenson, J., Aldington, S. *et al.* (1997). Retinopathy and vision loss in insulin dependent diabetes in Europe. The EURODIAB IDDM Complications Study. *Ophthalmology*, **104**, 252–60.

Stolk, R. P., Vingerling, J. R., de Jong, P. T. V. M. *et al.* (1995). Retinopathy, glucose and insulin in an elderly population. *Diabetes*, **44**, 11–15. The Rotterdam Study.

Sunness, J. S. (1998). The pregnant woman's eye. *Surv. Ophthalmol.*, **32**, 219–38.

The Diabetic Retinopathy Study Research Group (1979). Four risk factors for severe visual loss in diabetic retinopathy. The third report from the Diabetic Retinopathy Study. *Arch. Ophthalmol.*, **97**, 654–5.

The St Vincent Group (1990). Diabetes care and research in Europe. *Diab. Med.*, **7**, 360.

UK Prospective Diabetes Study Group (1998). Tight blood pressure control and risk of macrovascular complications in type 2 diabetes (UKPDS 38). *Br. Med. J.*, **317**, 713–20.

Von Jaeger, Q. E. (1856). *Beitraege zur Pathologie des Auges*. Wein.

Wilson, J. (1980). *World Blindness and its Prevention*, pp. 1–13. OUP.

Chapter 5

Features of diabetic eye disease
Gillian C. Vafidis

Introduction

The metabolic disturbances of diabetes affect all tissues. In the visual system the most obvious manifestation of diabetes is retinopathy, and a description of the features of diabetic retinopathy will form the main part of this chapter. In addition, diabetes is associated with ocular features such as cataract, glaucoma and neuropathy, and these features are discussed at the end of the chapter.

Features of diabetic retinopathy

Diabetic retinopathy primarily affects retinal capillaries. Although large retinal blood vessels are often abnormal in diabetes, this effect is secondary to the increased prevalence of hypertension and atherosclerosis, which cause arterial wall thickening and consequent venous changes. None of the individual features of diabetic retinopathy is unique to diabetes. However, the typical cluster of abnormal findings characteristically found together in diabetic retinopathy is highly suggestive of diabetes and often leads to the diagnosis in someone not previously known to be diabetic.

The development of retinopathy

The earliest ophthalmoscopic abnormalities of diabetic retinopathy are manifestations of increased capillary permeability. Exudates, haemorrhages and microaneurysms are easy to see on dilated retinal examination. With progression of retinopathy the features indicate retinal capillary closure and retinal ischaemia. These signs are more difficult to see. As closure becomes extensive, vasoproliferation in response to the retinal ischaemia occurs. In early proliferative disease these new vessels are difficult to detect on ophthalmoscopy, yet at this stage they are most readily treated. As they become more extensive, they are easier to diagnose and require much more aggressive treatment. As they grow into the vitreous cavity they give rise to the complications of vitreous haemorrhage and retinal traction, which are characteristic of advanced diabetic eye disease.

There is, therefore, a typical evolution of retinal features in diabetic retinopathy, with different lesions occurring at progressively more serious stages of severity. The stages are classified under four main headings, each representing groups of features that are characteristic of the stage:

1. Stage 1 – background diabetic retinopathy (also termed mild or moderate non-proliferative retinopathy)
2. Stage 2 – pre-proliferative diabetic retinopathy (also termed severe or very severe non-proliferative diabetic retinopathy)
3. Stage 3 – proliferative diabetic retinopathy (PDR)
4. Stage 4 – advanced diabetic eye disease, which is a term describing the sight-threatening complications of proliferative disease.

The features of each stage are summarized in Table 5.1.

Table 5.1 Summary of the features of diabetic retinopathy

Classification	Alternative terminology	Features
Background diabetic retinopathy	Mild/moderate non-proliferative diabetic retinopathy	Haemorrhages Oedema Microaneurysms Exudates Cotton wool spots Dilated veins
Pre-proliferative diabetic retinopathy	Severe/very severe non-proliferative retinopathy	Deep retinal haemorrhages in four quadrants Venous abnormalities Intraretinal microvascular abnormalities (IRMA) Multiple cotton wool spots
Proliferative diabetic retinopathy	Proliferative diabetic retinopathy (PDR)	New vessels on optic disc New vessels elsewhere
Advanced diabetic eye disease	Complications of proliferative diabetic retinopathy	Vitreous haemorrhage Retinal detachment Neovascular glaucoma

Background diabetic retinopathy

The dominant features of background diabetic retinopathy (BDR) reflect increased retinal capillary permeability. When these changes involve the macular capillaries, background retinopathy may affect vision directly and is termed maculopathy. The features of diabetic maculopathy are discussed at the end of this subsection.

The characteristic lesion of diabetic retinal capillary hyperpermeability is the microaneurysm. Leakage from microaneurysms causes retinal haemorrhages, oedema and exudates. In addition, cotton wool spots may be present, indicating microvascular occlusion in the nerve fibre layer with consequent swelling of the nerve axons. Dilated veins occur in BDR because of increased blood flow that is thought to be one of the consequences of hyperglycaemia. Characteristic patterns of background retinopathy are:

- circinate exudates surrounding a circle of oedema with central microaneurysm(s)
- cotton wool spots with flame haemorrhages and superficial retinal oedema.

The individual features will be discussed in detail.

Microaneurysms   Microaneurysms are an early feature of diabetic retinopathy (Figure 5.1). They represent a small weakness in the retinal capillary wall that leaks blood and serum. Their aetiology is not fully understood; they may represent an attempt to revascularize poorly perfused retina. They are seen as tiny red dots on ophthalmoscopy, and are often associated with a cap of retinal haemorrhage. They vary in size (10–100 μm in diameter), larger microaneurysms being surrounded by a circle of oedema, with hard exudates marking the boundary. Most microaneurysms are seen at the posterior pole, around the disc and macular area, where they may be the first ophthalmoscopic signs of diabetic retinopathy. In some cases they may be indistinguishable from small haemorrhages, and fluorescein angiography is needed to distinguish between these two features. They appear to come and go, becoming less visible as they thrombose, and with increasing capillary non-perfusion they may disappear entirely.

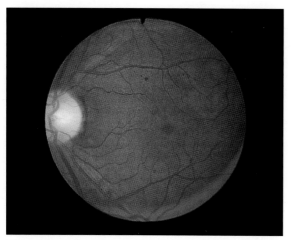
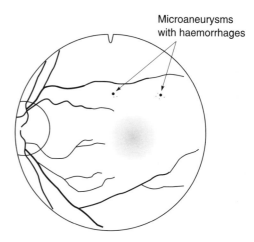

Figure 5.1 Microaneurysms in background diabetic retinopathy.

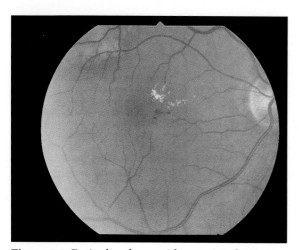
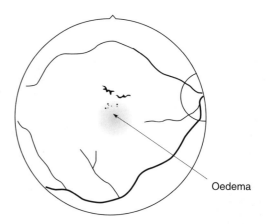

Figure 5.2 Retinal oedema with associated microaneurysms and exudates.

Oedema In diabetic retinopathy, oedema is caused by serum leaking into the retina through capillaries damaged by the changes of diabetes (Figure 5.2). Normally the retinal capillary wall forms an impermeable barrier between the bloodstream and retina. Diabetes damages that barrier, and allows blood and blood products to enter retinal tissue. As fluid accumulates, both within cells and within the extracellular space, retinal function may be disturbed. Disturbances to vision are more apparent to the patient the closer the oedema is to the fovea. If

the oedema affects the central fovea, it may cause permanent loss of vision.

Oedema is difficult to see on direct ophthalmoscopy because it is hard to appreciate retinal thickening without binocular clues. However, careful comparison with an adjacent area of retina may reveal a greyish blurring of deep retinal detail and a cystic appearance of the superficial retina in an area of oedema. It is useful to remember that where there are microaneurysms and exudates, there will be oedema. Using a binocular technique (e.g. using a 90 D

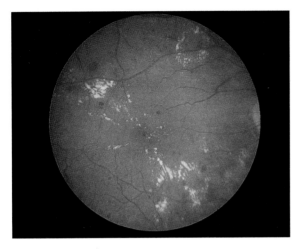

Figure 5.3 Exudates.

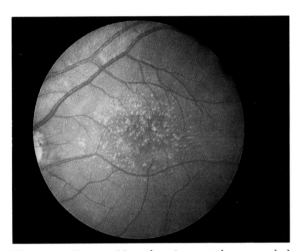

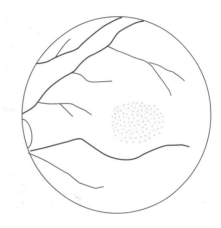

Figure 5.4 Drusen. Note the pigment clumps and absence of microaneurysms.

lens at the slit lamp), retinal oedema is more easily seen as retinal thickening.

Exudate Often described as hard exudates, these are deposits of extravasated plasma proteins, especially lipoproteins (Figure 5.3). They leak into retinal tissue with serum, and are left behind as oedema fluid is absorbed. Eventually exudates are cleared from the retina by macrophages.

On ophthalmoscopy, exudates are seen as yellow-white dots, flecks or plaques within the retina. They often appear shiny with sharp outlines. They are more commonly seen near the optic disc within the major blood vessel arcades, and cause sight loss if they impinge on the fovea. Exudates are easier to see than most other features of diabetic retinopathy, and even if the view is poor because of cataract they may be visible and indicate that, at the least, background diabetic retinopathy is present.

It is important to be able to distinguish exudates within the superficial retina from drusen beneath the neuroretina. Drusen (Figure

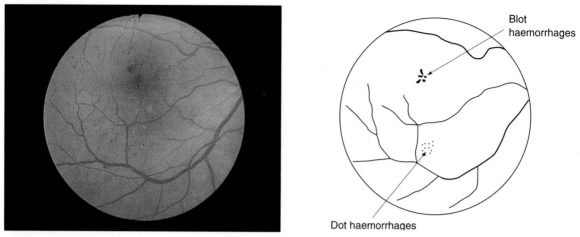

Figure 5.5 Haemorrhages in background diabetic retinopathy. They come in all shapes and sizes.

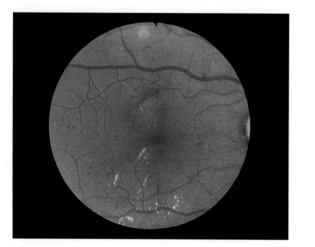
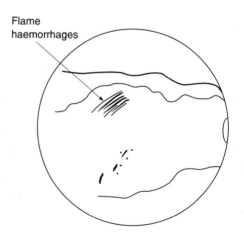

Figure 5.6 Flame haemorrhages. They lie along the nerve fibre layer and outline the direction of the fibres.

5.4) do not need referral to diabetic specialist centres, as they are manifestations of age-related macular degeneration (AMD) and are not in themselves sight-threatening. They may be of a similar shape and size to exudates, but usually have less distinct borders and are a pale, creamy yellow in colour. On biomicroscopy they can be seen to be at a deeper level of the retina and this is especially evident in areas where retinal vessels cross superficially to the drusen.

To help distinguish drusen from exudates, it is useful to remember that drusen are not associated with the other features of diabetic retinopathy – for example, microaneurysms. By contrast, they are associated with age-related macular changes of hypopigmentation and pigment clumping, are usually centred on the fovea and are often symmetrical between the two eyes.

Haemorrhages Intraretinal haemorrhages occur when blood leaks through damaged capillary walls into the retina, and they may be superficial or deep. On direct ophthalmoscopy, intraretinal haemorrhages are seen in three main forms – dot, blot or flame. Dot haemorrhages are indistinguishable from microaneurysms on fundoscopy, being tiny red spots within the superficial retina. Blot haemorrhages lie deeper. They are often larger, with irregular margins. Dark red blot haemorrhages may be retinal infarcts and they indicate retinal ischaemia (Figure 5.5). Flame haemorrhages are in the superficial retina and appear flame-shaped because the blood tracks in alignment with the superficial axons in the nerve fibre layer (Figure 5.6).

Cotton wool spots Cotton wool spots are common in background diabetic retinopathy (Figure 5.7). Each is caused by a small artery occlusion in the nerve fibre layer. Recent cotton wool spots are grey-white opaque patches in the superficial retina, aligned along the nerve fibre layer and often associated with small flame haemorrhages. As they age, cotton wool spots often whiten and may become stippled as tissue within them is cleared from the retina. Although cotton wool spots are frequently found in early retinopathy, large numbers of them throughout the retina indicate widespread ischaemia. They may be an important sign of more advanced and rapidly progressing retinopathy, as may occur in pregnancy and when high blood sugar is brought under control rapidly.

Large numbers of cotton wool spots are also characteristic of large vessel disease and are seen in accelerated hypertension, even without accompanying diabetic retinopathy.

Dilated retinal veins Dilation of the principal retinal veins indicates early diabetic retinopathy, and it may be present before any other diabetic retinopathy develops (Figure 5.8). It is often not an obvious feature and is difficult to appreciate on ophthalmoscopy. It is thought to indicate increased blood flow which is related to hyperglycaemia and reduced vascular tone.

Maculopathy – BDR at the macula

Maculopathy is background retinopathy within the macular area, i.e. within a two disc diameter radius of the centre of the fovea. It is classified as oedematous or ischaemic, though the two types frequently coexist.

In oedematous maculopathy, macular oedema causes visual problems because of capillary leakage. The oedema is either focal, where it is localized to discrete areas within the macula, or diffuse, affecting the entire macular area.

In ischaemic maculopathy, capillary closure causes loss of vision by affecting the perfusion of the central fovea.

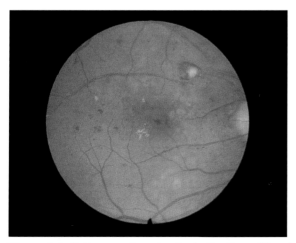
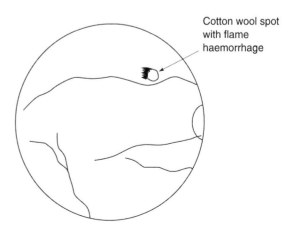

Cotton wool spot with flame haemorrhage

Figure 5.7 Cotton wool spots. An indication of local arteriolar occlusion.

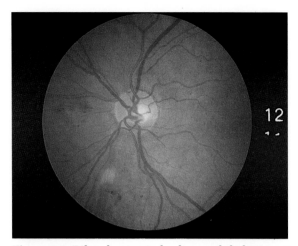

Dilated
vein

Figure 5.8 Dilated veins in background diabetic retinopathy.

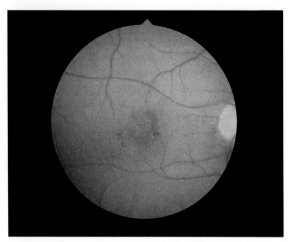

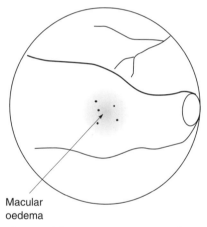

Macular
oedema

Figure 5.9 Macular oedema. Note the grey colour of the retinal oedema with microaneurysms and haemorrhages close by.

Macular oedema Macular oedema is defined as an area of retinal thickening within the macular area (Figure 5.9). It can involve all (diffuse) or part (focal) of the macular area. Focal macular oedema is often associated with normal vision.

It may be difficult to see macular oedema with a direct ophthalmoscope. If it involves the central area there is loss of the foveal reflex, often with an apparent increase in yellow pigment and an associated reduction in visual acuity. Sometimes it is possible to appreciate the petalloid appearance of superficial retinal cysts in diffuse cystoid macular oedema. Focal oedema can be appreciated as a patch of grey retina with central microaneurysms and surrounding exudates (circinate pattern). On binocular examination, retinal thickening involving the fovea is seen.

'Clinically significant macular oedema' (CSMO) is a term used to identify patterns of macular oedema which will result in significant visual loss if not treated with laser photocoagulation of the underlying pigment epithelium (ETDRS, 1985). Any of the following characteristics are defined as CSMO:

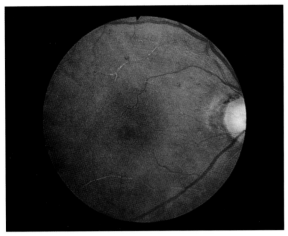 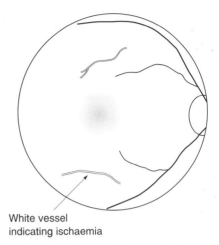

White vessel
indicating ischaemia

Figure 5.10 Macular ischaemia. The retina looks dark and white blood vessels pass close to the foveal area, indicating capillary closure.

- retinal thickening within 500 μm of the fovea
- exudates within 500 μm of the fovea
- an area of retinal thickening larger than one disc area, any part of which is within one disc diameter of the fovea.

This definition is used by ophthalmologists when deciding upon treatment. A distance of 500 μm is approximately equivalent to one-third of the disc diameter. The former method of quantifying distance is preferred to the latter, because optic discs vary in size between individuals.

Macular ischaemia Macular ischaemia is a result of closure of the capillaries normally supplying the foveal arcade (Figure 5.10). It is impossible to diagnose with certainty on ophthalmoscopy. Features suggesting blood vessel closure include the presence of dilated retinal capillaries or white vessels near the macula. Often a subtle change in appearance of the underlying pigment epithelium occurs in an area of capillary closure. In addition, there may be unexplained poor vision when closure involves the perifoveal arcade. The diagnosis is made on fundus fluorescein angiography.

Features of pre-proliferative diabetic retinopathy

The features of pre-proliferative retinopathy have been found to be associated with an increased risk of the development of proliferative retinopathy. Pre-proliferative disease is a response to retinal capillary closure.

Intraretinal microvascular abnormalities Intraretinal microvascular abnormalities (IRMA) are fine intraretinal blood vessels that grow within retinal tissue (Figure 5.11). They usually originate from the venous side of the retinal circulation and grow towards an area of capillary closure. It is thought that they represent an attempt to revascularize ischaemic retina. Although they are new vessels, they do not bleed or cause preretinal or vitreous haemorrhage. On fluorescein angiography only the growing tips leak dye, in contrast to proliferative new vessels. IRMA can be distinguished from normal retinal blood vessels by their haphazard branching, with unusually large angles between branches and an irregular calibre that varies from fine thread-like vessels to dilated capillaries in the same IRMA. IRMA are most commonly seen within an area five

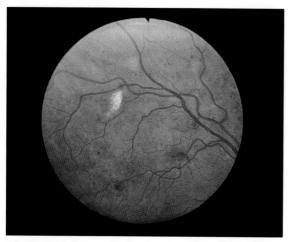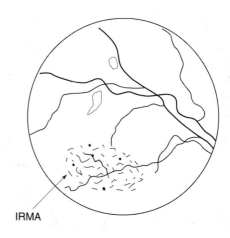

Figure 5.11 Intraretinal microvascular abnormalities (IRMA). Note the haphazard appearance and calibre of intraretinal microvascular abnormalities.

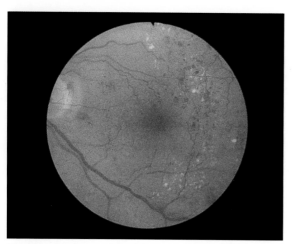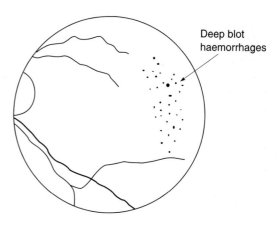

Figure 5.12 Deep retinal haemorrhages. They indicate ischaemia and are commonly found temporal to the macula.

disc diameters around the optic disc between major blood vessels. Because they are intra-retinal, they never overlie the major vessels. A significant area of IRMA represents a four-fold increased risk of proliferative retinopathy developing within a year.

Deep retinal haemorrhages The presence of widespread intraretinal haemorrhages in the four quadrants of the retina indicates a four-fold increased risk of proliferative retinopathy appearing within a year (Figure 5.12). When retinal haemorrhages appear dark they represent retinal ischaemia, and are characteristically found temporal to the macula.

Venous abnormalities The presence of venous abnormalities affecting the large retinal veins is a powerful predictor of proliferative retinopathy developing within a year (Figure 5.13). Pre-proliferative venous changes include variations in calibre and abnormal looping and doubling. The calibre changes occur as a vein crosses an area of retinal ischaemia. It may

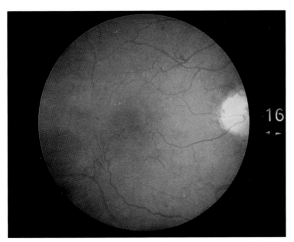
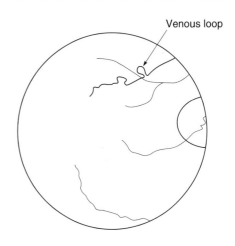

Figure 5.13 Venous abnormalities. Loops and calibre changes indicate retinal ischaemia and an increased risk of proliferative retinopathy.

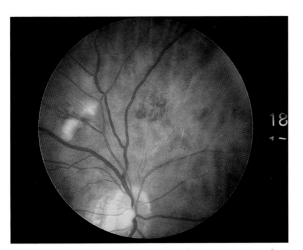
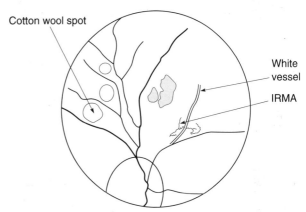

Figure 5.14 Multiple cotton wool spots. May indicate retinal ischaemia, especially if associated with other pre-proliferative features.

appear to take on the appearance of a string of sausages, with localized constrictions and dilations. Sometimes normal flow can be seen to resume more peripherally in the same vessel if the surrounding retina is less ischaemic.

Venous loops and doubling occur because of recanalization of the vein after partial occlusion. Doubling represents the development of collateral channels.

Multiple cotton wool spots Large numbers of cotton wool spots are an indication of sig-

nificant retinal ischaemia (Figure 5.14). When found in association with moderate background features, they represent a doubling of the risk of proliferative retinopathy developing within a year.

Proliferative diabetic retinopathy

Proliferative disease is the most serious treatable stage of diabetic retinopathy. If adequate laser treatment can be given before advanced disease develops, visual loss can be prevented.

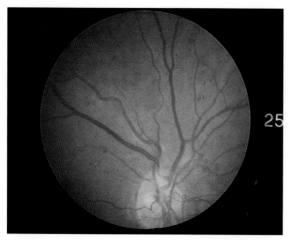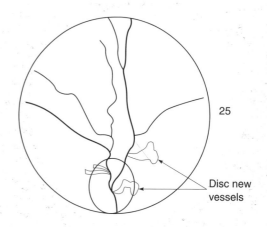

Figure 5.15 Disc new vessels. Note how fine early disc new vessels are compared with normal retinal vessels.

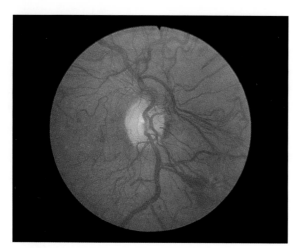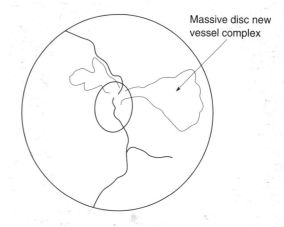

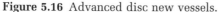
Figure 5.16 Advanced disc new vessels.

In proliferative disease, new blood vessels grow forwards from large retinal veins towards the vitreous. They are stimulated to grow by the release of growth factors by ischaemic retina. New vessels represent a serious threat to vision because they bleed, causing vitreous and pre-retinal haemorrhages. In addition, fibrous tissue growing forwards with the new vessels can be responsible for traction on the retina, which may cause macular retinal detachment.

Proliferative new vessels arise either from veins on the optic disc or from more peripheral large veins.

Disc new vessels New vessels arising from the disc (NVD) carry a major risk of blindness if left untreated (Figure 5.15). Recognizing disc new vessels on ophthalmoscopy is not easy when they are early in their development. At this stage they are fine and wispy, with a single origin from a large vein. The stalk of the new vessel often quickly divides into fine random branches that extend into the vitreous gel, the growing tips angulated away from each other. If not treated at this stage, the new vessels become sturdier and the new vessel complex becomes larger (Fig 5.16). Prevention

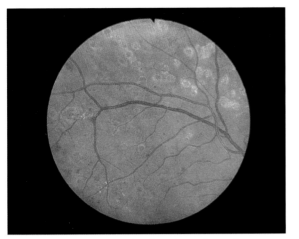
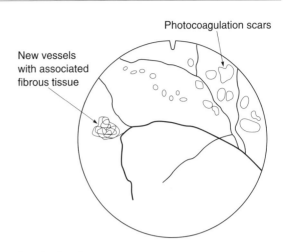

Figure 5.17 New vessels elsewhere from the superotemporal retinal vein.

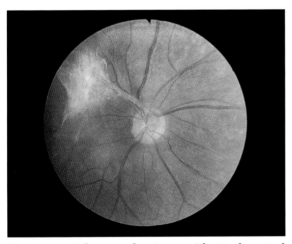
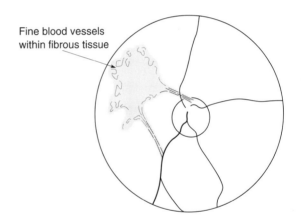

Figure 5.18 Fibrovascular tissue with attachments between disc and superotemporal vessels.

of haemorrhagic or tractional complications becomes more difficult the more extensive the new vessel, and it is essential that early proliferative retinopathy is detected and referred for treatment.

New vessels elsewhere New vessels elsewhere (NVE) are proliferative new vessels that grow from large retinal veins (Figure 5.17). The new vessel stalk often arises from a bifurcation in a main vein and quickly forms a network of branches. NVE can be distinguished from IRMA (intraretinal new vessels) because they

arise from and may overlie main vessels. Uncomplicated NVE carry less risk of blindness than disc new vessels. However, studies have shown that once NVE are associated with vitreous haemorrhage, significant visual loss occurs if they are not treated promptly with laser panretinal photocoagulation. Up to one-third of patients with NVE will develop disc new vessels within a year.

Fibrovascular tissue As new vessels grow they are supported by fibrous tissue produced by retinal glial cells. The fibrous tissue appears white on ophthalmoscopy, and in some patients may be more apparent than the new vessels themselves (Figure 5.18). Fibrous tissue is often seen in association with NVE, where the new vessel arises from the veins of the major arcades. The danger of the fibrous tissue is that sooner or later it contracts, causing bleeding of the new vessels (vitreous and preretinal haemorrhage) and traction on the new vessel stalk. The traction may lift the retina away from the pigment epithelium and its blood supply into the vitreous cavity, causing retinal folds and traction retinal detachment. If traction involves the macula, vision will be affected. Alternatively, if the retina does not detach, where fibrous tissue is firmly adherent to the retina and contracts it may tear a retinal hole.

The consequences and complications of proliferative retinopathy

Retinal laser burns

It is important to be able to recognize laser scars and to distinguish them from other possible causes of retinal pigmentation (Fig. 7.2). There are two main patterns of retinal laser scars, macular treatment and peripheral scatter treatment, and these are discussed in more detail under treatment in Chapter 7.

Advanced diabetic eye disease

Advanced disease arises as a complication of the fibrovascular response to retinal ischaemia. Recent improvements in treatment techniques mean that advanced disease is not inevitably associated with loss of vision, but the chances of maintaining normal vision are poor once advanced disease develops.

Vitreous haemorrhage Vitreous haemorrhage may obscure all view of the retina, and it should always be assumed that proliferative diabetic retinopathy has developed when vitreous haemorrhage develops in a diabetic patient. The haemorrhage is sometimes confined between the vitreous gel and retinal surface, and this is called a preretinal haemorrhage (Figure 5.19). A preretinal haemorrhage typically forms horizontal fluid levels, often inferotemporal to the optic disc, and may obscure the macula, making the site of the proliferative vessel causing the bleeding difficult to see.

Epiretinal fibrosis and traction Contraction of fibrovascular tissue resulting from proliferative disease may exert traction on the retina (Figure. 5.20). Traction retinal detachment appears as a concave greyish elevation, which is often localized, and causes visual loss if it involves the

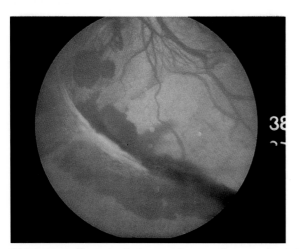
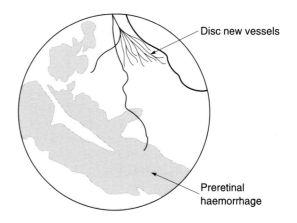

Figure 5.19 Preretinal vitreous haemorrhage in the inferior retina caused by bleeding from disc new vessels.

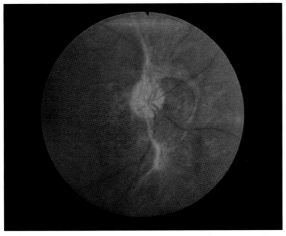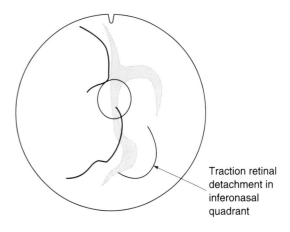

Traction retinal
detachment in
inferonasal
quadrant

Figure 5.20 Fibrovascular traction and tractional retinal detachment.

macula. In some cases vitreous traction is complicated by retinal hole formation, and total retinal detachment may result.

Iris new vessels and neovascular glaucoma
With extensive retinal ischaemia and the consequent production of neovascular growth factors, new blood vessels develop on the iris and in the drainage angle of the front of the eye (rubeosis iridis). The fibrous tissue that accompanies the new blood vessels closes the angle, and this results in secondary (neovascular) glaucoma. Treatment options are few, and are often unsuccessful in retaining sight. It is usually possible to prevent the blind eye becoming painful and needing removal by performing retinal and ciliary body ablation with laser or cryotherapy.

Neovascular glaucoma is an uncommon complication of diabetic retinopathy, occurring after the development of retinal new vessels. If adequate treatment for retinal ischaemia can be given in time, early iris new vessels regress and glaucoma does not develop.

Non-retinal diabetic ocular disease

Diabetes affects every cell in the body, and it is not surprising that there is an increased incidence of other ocular pathology in diabetes.

Cataract The most common non-retinal finding in diabetes is the accelerated appearance of age-related lens changes. Diabetes is a strong risk factor for cataract, especially in women.

Rarely, cortical cataract can be the transient result of changes in blood sugar level and is most common in Type 1 diabetes. These lens opacities usually clear with stabilization of control.

Permanent early cortical snowflake lens opacities can develop in both Type 1 and Type 2 diabetes. Although similar lens opacities may be induced experimentally by changes in osmolality, the cause of diabetic cataract in humans is thought to be linked to abnormal levels of antioxidants and to be an exacerbation of age-related cataract. In diabetic patients cataract begins earlier and progresses at a faster rate than in the general population, and is more prevalent in Afro-Caribbean and Asian populations.

Cataract surgery is often more difficult in diabetic patients. The iris does not dilate fully and the immediate post-operative course may be complicated by a higher incidence of inflammation. Late post-operative complications include a reported higher incidence of posterior capsule opacification. Cataract surgery has also been reported to be associated with rapid progression of retinopathy, and for this reason cataract surgery is contraindicated unless prior laser treatment has been given to stabilize retinopathy.

Glaucoma Recent epidemiological studies have confirmed the association between diabetes and an increased risk of glaucoma and raised intraocular pressure (Mitchell *et al.*, 1997; Dielemans *et al.*, 1996). Abnormal glycoprotein deposition in the iris in diabetes may affect pupil size and shape and alter aqueous drainage channels. Diabetic neuropathy can involve the autonomic nervous system of the iris, and may be linked with intraocular pressure changes in diabetes. Where glaucoma is present, diabetic changes in the retinal circulation may make glaucomatous optic disc damage more likely in diabetic patients than in those with a healthy retinal blood supply.

Cranial nerve palsy Diabetic microvascular disease may affect small vessels supplying the motor cranial nerves. The sixth cranial nerve supplying the lateral rectus muscle is most commonly affected. The diabetic patient (usually Type 2) presents with sudden onset of horizontal double vision on looking towards the affected side. On examination, the affected eye is unable to move laterally. It is usual for diabetic sixth nerve palsy to recover, with gradual return of lateral rectus function over a few months. Diabetes-related third nerve palsy is also well recognized, and is characteristically pupil sparing – in other words, although the third nerve supplies the autonomic nerve fibres responsible for pupil constriction, when third nerve palsy is due to diabetes these fibres are not involved and the pupil constricts normally. In third nerve palsy the patient may present with a unilateral ptosis and involvement of the muscles of upgaze and adduction. The natural history is one of recovery of full function in the majority of cases.

Retinal vascular disease The incidence of retinal vascular disease is higher in diabetes, even without diabetic retinopathy, because of the atherogenic effect of diabetes on the large retinal arteries. Increased rigidity and thickness of retinal arterial walls is also caused by hypertension, which is more common in diabetes. The venous return is compromised where an artery crosses a vein. Initially, arteriovenous nipping and increased tortuosity are seen. If retinal venous flow is severely compromised, retinal vein occlusion occurs.

At the optic disc, involvement of the arterial supply to the optic nerve results in ischaemic optic neuropathy, which is more common in diabetes.

Other effects of diabetes

- Vitreous opacity. Asteroid hyalitis is more common in diabetes. The vitreous gel has a diffuse infiltration of shiny pale opacities that vary in size and are made up of deposits of lipoproteins, especially cholesterol.
- Infections. Diabetes is associated with relative immune suppression. This means that there is an increased susceptibility to infection and poorer wound healing. Tissue repair may be slow and be complicated by secondary infection.

Ocular conditions that protect from retinopathy

The serious effects of diabetic eye disease are caused by retinal ischaemia. Conditions in which there is little metabolic activity in the retina therefore have a reduced incidence of diabetic retinopathy, even after many years of the disease. In high myopia and advanced glaucoma where extensive retinal atrophy occurs, it is well recognized that diabetic retinopathy may not occur to the same degree as where retinal tissue is healthy. It has been suggested that amblyopia affords relative protection from severe diabetic retinopathy, although there are many clinical examples of advanced diabetic eye disease in amblyopia.

In summary, it is unwise to assume that any

diabetic eye is safe from retinopathy. Asymmetry and lack of symptoms in diabetic eye disease are well recognized. Normal visual acuity may coexist with proliferative diabetic retinopathy. Alongside advances in the treatment of diabetic retinopathy, the single most important factor in preventing blindness is retinal examination of every diabetic person to identify features of diabetic retinopathy.

References

Dielemans, I., de Jong, P. T., Stolk, R. *et al.*, (1996). Primary open angle glaucoma, intraocular pressure and diabetes mellitus in the general elderly population. The Rotterdam Study. *Ophthalmology*, **103**, 1271–5.

Early Treatment Diabetic Retinopathy Study Group (1985). Report No. 1. Photocoagulation for diabetic macular oedema. *Arch. Ophthalmol.*, **103**, 1796–1806.

Mitchell, P., Smith, W., Chey, T. and Healey, P. R. (1997). Open angle glaucoma and diabetes: the Blue Mountain eye study, Australia. *Ophthalmology*, **104**, 712–18.

Further reading

Hamilton, A. M. P., Ulbig, M. W. and Polkinghorne, P. (1996). *Management of Diabetic Retinopathy*. BMJ Publishing Group.

Chapter 6

Management of diabetic retinopathy: criteria for referral and management of the post-laser patient

Paul Sullivan

Introduction

The natural history of diabetic retinopathy is of progression through several stages. These run from no diabetic retinopathy through mild asymptomatic disease (at which stage treatment is not required) and more severe asymptomatic disease (at which stage treatment is best carried out) to advanced retinopathy characterized by visual impairment and a less satisfactory response to treatment.

The general principle in deciding when to refer a diabetic patient for further assessment by an ophthalmologist is to allow effective treatment to be carried out with the best chance of a good visual outcome. There is no general consensus on the ideal stage at which referral

should be made. The referral criteria in this chapter are based on those used in screening programmes with which Moorfields Eye Hospital is involved. Screening programmes used elsewhere may use different referral criteria. The urgency of referral is determined by the speed of progression of the untreated disease.

Stage of retinopathy and referral

Table 6.1 summarizes the stages of retinopathy and referral criteria.

No diabetic retinopathy

The probability of progressing to sight-threatening retinopathy within 12 months is

Table 6.1 Stage of retinopathy and summary of referral criteria

Examination findings	Action
No retinopathy	Review 12 months
Background diabetic retinopathy	Review 6 months
Diabetic maculopathy	Refer soon (within 8 weeks)
Pre-proliferative diabetic retinopathy	Refer soon (within 8 weeks)
Mild proliferative diabetic retinopathy	Refer soon (within 8 weeks)
Severe proliferative diabetic retinopathy	Refer urgently (2 weeks)
Advanced diabetic retinopathy	Refer urgently (2 weeks)
Inadequate fundal view	Refer (see text)
Unattributable loss of central vision	Refer soon (within 8 weeks)

extremely low, and a further examination should therefore be scheduled for 12 months hence.

Background diabetic retinopathy

Background diabetic retinopathy is defined by the presence of microaneurysms anywhere in the retina and/or exudates or haemorrhages not nearer than one disc-diameter from the fovea (i.e. any retinopathy not sufficiently severe to qualify for one of the categories given below).

These patients should be reviewed by the optometrist at 6-month intervals.

Diabetic maculopathy

Diabetic maculopathy (Whitelock *et al.*, 1985) is clearly described in Chapter 5, and the features of diabetic maculopathy outlined below relate to the referral criteria recommended in this chapter.

The presence of microaneurysms alone within one disc diameter of the fovea does not automatically qualify the patient for referral, provided that the examiner has the ability to exclude retinal thickening (macular oedema) in these patients using slit lamp biomicroscopy. If this is not possible (for example, if examination is being carried out with a direct ophthalmoscope alone), then patients with microaneurysms alone within a disc diameter of the fovea should be referred. These patients should be referred to an ophthalmologist soon (ideally within 8 weeks).

Note that although early referral is suggested, this is not urgent; the Early Treatment Diabetic Retinopathy Study Group (1985) showed that visual loss in maculopathy occurs over a period of months. Hard exudates 'threatening' fixation do not do so at the same rate or have the same urgency as a retinal detachment.

Note: The definition of maculopathy used here does not coincide with that used in the Early Treatment Diabetic Retinopathy Study Group (1985) of clinically significant macular oedema, where it was defined as any of the following characteristics:

- retinal thickening within 500 µm of the fovea
- exudates within 500 µm of the fovea
- an area of retinal thickening larger than one disc area, any part of which is within one disc diameter of the fovea.

(NB: 500 µm is approximately one-third of the disc diameter.)

This latter definition is the one used by most ophthalmologists to determine the presence of threshold disease requiring laser treatment. The simpler definition advocated here will cause some over-referral, but these are eyes at significant risk of developing sight-threatening retinopathy and it is appropriate that they should be monitored by an ophthalmologist. It is worth noting that the presence of normal visual acuity should not deter one from referring these patients, as sight-threatening retinopathy may still be present and it is at this stage that treatment has most benefit.

Pre-proliferative retinopathy

Proliferative retinopathy is defined by the presence of extensive haemorrhages, multiple cotton wool spots (one or two cotton wool spots do not have the same significance), abnormalities of retinal veins ('beading' and 'reduplication') and intraretinal microvascular anomalies (IRMA). A detailed description of these anomalies is given in Chapter 5. These lesions indicate a very ischaemic retina which is at a high risk of progressing to sight-threatening retinopathy. Early referral to an ophthalmologist is recommended (ideally within 8 weeks).

Mild proliferative retinopathy

Mild proliferative retinopathy is defined by the presence of retinal new vessels more than one disc diameter away from the disc in the absence of preretinal or vitreous haemorrhage (see Chapter 5). The risk of visual loss in the short term is relatively low, and no benefit of treatment was shown by the Diabetic Retinopathy Study Research Group (1976, 1981). However, because progression to high-risk retinopathy is usual, most British ophthalmologists now carry out retinal photocoagulation in these cases. Early referral to an ophthalmologist is recommended (ideally within 8 weeks).

Severe proliferative retinopathy

Severe proliferative retinopathy is defined by the presence of retinal new vessels on the optic disc or bleeding new vessels away from the disc. This is the group with the highest rate of visual loss (Diabetic Retinopathy Study Research Group, 1981). Prompt retinal photocoagulation is indicated in these patients, and they should therefore be referred to an ophthalmologist urgently (ideally within 2 weeks). The rationale behind the urgency in this group is that vitreous haemorrhage occurring prior to review in the eye clinic may make treatment difficult or necessitate an early vitrectomy.

Any health professional involved in screening will be anxious about the possibility of overlooking some serious abnormality. It is in this group of patients with severe proliferative diabetic retinopathy that the consequences of overlooking the pathology will be most serious. Early disc new vessels may easily be overlooked, so it is always worth paying special attention to the optic disc while screening.

Advanced diabetic retinopathy

The hallmark of this group is the presence of a fibrous reaction on the surfaces of the retina and vitreous to the presence of blood and new vessel complexes. This process, and not blood in the vitreous *per se*, is now the major cause of severe visual loss in diabetic patients. The fibrous tissue contracts, pulling the retina into folds and detaching it. These patients should therefore be referred to an ophthalmologist urgently (ideally within 2 weeks).

Inadequate fundal view

This is usually due to a combination of cataract and poorly dilating pupils. Sometimes a reasonable view of the fundus is possible using a slit lamp. If the view of the retina is not adequate for screening, then a cataract extraction may be necessary to monitor the retina.

These patients should be referred on a routine basis for hospital screening, provided there is no history of sudden visual loss.

A less common cause is vitreous haemorrhage from bleeding new vessel complexes. Such patients give a history of acute visual loss and, provided the problem is not bilateral, have marked retinopathy in the fellow eye. These patients should therefore be referred to an ophthalmologist urgently (ideally within 2 weeks).

Loss of central vision

A list of some of the more common causes of attributable loss of central vision in a diabetic patient is given in Table 6.2.

The osmotic effects of fluctuating blood glucose on the lens, causing unstable refractive state, are well known to optometrists. A thorough optometric examination should exclude this as a possible cause of visual loss by demonstrating improvement in vision with a change of spectacle correction.

Epidemiological studies have shown cataract to be the most common cause of mildly reduced vision (to approximately 6/18) in diabetic patients.

Glaucoma and age-related macular degeneration are important causes of visual loss in diabetic patients, as they are in the general population.

Where there is no attributable cause of central visual loss, patients should be referred

Table 6.2 Common causes of visual loss in diabetic patients

- Altered refraction (compounded by fluctuating blood glucose)
- Cataract
- Vitreous haemorrhage
- Tractional retinal detachment
- Glaucoma
- Maculopathy
- Age-related macular degeneration
- Ischaemic optic neuropathy
- Diabetic papillopathy
- Cerebrovascular disease

to an ophthalmologist soon (ideally within 8 weeks).

When to re-refer

There are three scenarios in which an optometrist may consider re-referring a patient who has previously been referred to an eye department.

1. The patient has been seen and discharged from the eye clinic. The fact that the patient was previously seen and given the 'all clear' some time previously does not mean that he or she does not need to be seen again. The situation may have changed during the intervening period. The referral criteria in this instance are identical to those laid down in the earlier part of this chapter.
2. The patient is still under review by the eye clinic. In most instances this occurs because a patient requires a refraction. Optometrists are in a difficult position when examining patients who are receiving continuing care in an eye clinic. They are under a contractual obligation to notify the general practitioner of any abnormality that they detect on examination, while both the GP and the hospital are aware that the patient has significant retinopathy. A letter merely informing the GP of action taken should be sufficient in most cases, and re-referral to the clinic shouldn't be necessary.
3. An alternative scenario to that above is one of shared care for the diabetic patient. Here the optometrist would be involved not only in screening but also in the supervision of the patient after treatment. Such shared care schemes have been advocated in the management of glaucoma, and are almost routine in the aftercare of patients who have undergone cataract surgery. Their application in diabetic retinopathy may be more problematic. The ability to detect significant pathology in an eye that has already received treatment and to determine the need for retreatment is necessary. This is much more complicated than screening, but may be an option in the future. On the assumption that

the role of the optometrist could theoretically be extended in this direction, a brief account of how this is done follows.

Optometric surveillance: assessing the effects of treatment

After successful laser treatment for proliferative diabetic retinopathy, new vessels undergo a set of changes called 'regression'. New vessel complexes that are wide in the active phase of the disease become thin and wispy, and a small amount of fibrous tissue often forms around them as this happens. This process usually occurs within 8 weeks of treatment. Other changes in the retina indicate the adequacy of treatment. Retinal veins, which are often widely dilated in proliferative diabetic retinopathy because of inner retinal hypoxia, return to a normal calibre or become thinner than usual. Panretinal photocoagulation normalizes the concentration of oxygen in the inner retina, and is believed to be responsible for the observed change in retinal veins. Neovascular complexes should not develop in new locations if the laser treatment was adequate.

The response of diabetic maculopathy to photocoagulation is often more difficult to assess. 'Focal' laser treatment, in which the laser is applied to isolated leaking areas surrounded by exudates (so called 'circinate' lesions), is often dramatically successful in eliminating the exudates and maintaining good vision. The exudates take some months to resolve, but as long as all the leaking areas have been treated no further treatment is required. The response of 'diffuse' diabetic maculopathy is more difficult to assess. Here the leakage into the retina is more widespread, and treatment consists of a 'grid' of laser burns in the leaking areas. Gauging the response to treatment depends on the ability to assess retinal thickening using stereo biomicroscopy. Such patients often require more than one session of laser treatment.

Patients who have received retinal photocoagulation invariably need lifelong follow-up. Patients who have been lost to follow-up after undergoing photocoagulation for diabetic retinopathy should always be referred back to an eye clinic.

Optometric management of the post-laser patient

Apart from assessing diabetic retinopathy, several points need to be borne in mind by the optometrist seeing patients after retinal photocoagulation. The patient may have unusual visual problems attributable to diabetic retinopathy or to retinal laser treatment or to a combination of the two. In addition, diabetic patients may have special visual needs that the optometrist should be aware of.

Visual problems after retinal laser photocoagulation

Retinal photocoagulation has dramatically improved the outlook for patients with diabetic retinopathy (Klein and Klein, 1992). Even after successful photocoagulation, patients may have visual problems. While most of these are due to the underlying disease, some are a direct consequence of the treatment and have to be regarded as the price to be paid for avoiding total blindness.

Although patients with widespread retinal ischaemia often have peripheral scotomas, they are unlikely to be symptomatic. Destruction of peripheral retina by extensive panretinal photocoagulation may cause night blindness and peripheral visual field defects that may be severe enough to prohibit driving. Damage to the long ciliary nerves may interfere with accommodation and cause early presbyopia. Patients may also show abnormalities in tests of colour vision and contrast sensitivity. Colour vision defects may interfere with patients' ability to use BM stix to monitor their blood glucose (see below).

Laser treatment using a contact lens very occasionally results in corneal abrasions, which tend to be slow to heal in diabetic patients.

Severe visual loss is relatively uncommon after photocoagulation. Visual acuity may fall after macular photocoagulation due to inadvertent photocoagulation of the fovea. Patients with very aggressive proliferative retinopathy sometimes suffer vitreous haemorrhages after panretinal photocoagulation. Such haemorrhages are as much a reflection of the severity of the disease as a complication of the treatment, but patients may understandably be bitter if their vision is affected.

Managing the visually impaired diabetic patient

Visually impaired diabetic patients have many of the same visual needs as non-diabetic patients. Thus they may benefit from the standard supportive measures such as advice on lighting, visual aids and blind or partial sight registration. However, their ability to cope with blindness may be reduced by their diabetes – for example, peripheral neuropathy causes reduced ability to feel with the tips of the fingers and can make it difficult to read Braille. Some patients may manage better with another type of language such as Moon.

Diabetic patients often test their own blood at home using BM stix. This involves putting a little drop of their blood on a little plastic strip and observing a colour change in the strip. This may be difficult either because of impaired visual acuity or colour vision deficits. One solution is to advise patients to use a meter that reads the colour change and has a large, high-contrast digital read out.

Diabetic patients who require insulin have to draw up the amount to be given very exactly in a syringe. Many patients find this difficult as it involves watching the movement of the syringe plunger against a very fine scale on the wall of the syringe. Previously, syringes with devices to stop movement of the plunger were used to allow the patient to draw up the correct amount of insulin. Now a device such as the Novopen™ is often used. This pen-like tool contains a cartridge of insulin and expresses a small amount of insulin each time a button on the end is pressed. The amount of insulin given is gauged by the number of clicks.

Table 6.3 Special visual needs of diabetic patients

Problem	Solution
Unable to see to draw up insulin	Novopen
Unable to see to cut toenails	Refer to chiropodist
Unable to read blood glucose monitoring strips	Use digital or talking meter

Diabetic patients may suffer severe complications after even minor trauma to their feet. It is therefore advisable for patients with poor vision to consider arranging for a chiropodist to cut their toenails.

The special visual needs of diabetic patients are summarized in Table 6.3.

Despite the advances in the management of patients with diabetes over the last 30 years, diabetic retinopathy remains the most common cause of blindness in people of working age in the United Kingdom. The consequences of visual loss in diabetic patients are thus particularly severe, and knowledge of this should make all healthcare professionals dealing with diabetic patients redouble their efforts to prevent it.

References

Diabetic Retinopathy Study Research Group (1976). Preliminary report on the effects of photocoagulation therapy. *Am. J. Ophthalmol.*, **81**, 383–96.

Diabetic Retinopathy Study Research Group (1981). Photocoagulation treatment of proliferative diabetic retinopathy. DRS report number 8. *Ophthamology*, **88**, 583–600.

Early Treatment Diabetic Retinopathy Study Group (1985). Report No. 1. Photocoagulation for diabetic macular oedema. *Arch. Ophthalmol.*, **103**, 1796–1806.

Klein, R. and Klein, B. E. K. (1992). Visual impairment and diabetes. In: *International Textbook of Diabetes Mellitus* (K. G. M. Alberti, R. A. Defronzo, H. Keen and P. Zimmet, eds), pp. 1373–85. Wiley and Sons.

Whitelocke, R. A. F., Kearns, M., Blach, R. K. and Hamilton, A. M. (1979). The diabetic maculopathies. *Trans. Ophthalmol. Soc. UK*, **99**, 314–20.

Further reading

Kraws, H. M. J., Porta, M. and Keen, H. (1990). A protocol for screening for diabetic retinopathy in Europe. In: *Diabetes Care and Research in Europe: The St Vincent Declaration Action Programme* (H. M. J. Kraws, ed.). World Health Organisation.

Sonksen, P., Fox, C. and Judd, S. (1986). *The Diabetes Reference Book*. Harper and Row.

Chapter 7

Treatment of diabetic retinopathy
G. W. Aylward

This chapter will outline methods used for the treatment of diabetic retinopathy, but it would be incomplete without a brief mention of the importance of good systemic control of diabetes.

Tight diabetic control

The normal pancreas maintains very close control over the level of circulating glucose. It achieves this by means of a negative feedback loop similar to the operation of a thermostat in a central heating system. If the level of blood glucose rises, for example following a meal, the islet cells in the pancreas are stimulated to release more insulin. Insulin acts so as to reduce the level of circulating glucose. If the glucose level falls, then the islet cells produce less insulin, allowing the glucose level to stabilize.

This tight feedback cannot be matched by intermittent injections of insulin in patients with diabetes, and it is inevitable that there will be abnormally wide fluctuations in glucose level. To return to the analogy with a central heating system, controlling diabetes with twice daily injections of insulin is akin to controlling the house temperature by having an engineer visit twice a day to adjust the controls.

Patients with diabetes are at risk of developing a series of long-term complications. These include cardiovascular disease, renal problems, neuropathy and, of course, retinopathy. There is compelling evidence that these complications are related directly to elevated glucose levels. Studies in animals have shown that tighter control reduces the risk of long-term complications from diabetes. It was always assumed that the same applied to humans, although direct clinical evidence had to await the publication of the Diabetes Control and Complications Trial in 1993. This was a large randomized controlled trial in 1441 patients with diabetes. Patients were randomized to receive either conventional treatment, with one or two daily injections of insulin, or intensive treatment consisting of three or more injections and multiple blood glucose monitoring. The results were positive, with the risk of developing retinopathy over a 6-year period being reduced by 76 per cent in the intensive therapy group.

Retinal photocoagulation

One of the first major insights into the treatment of proliferative diabetic retinopathy was provided by Poulsen's observation in 1953. He observed that pituitary infarction due to postpartum haemorrhage in a diabetic patient with severe proliferative diabetic retinopathy led to regression of the new vessels. Pituitary ablation by surgery or radioactive yttrium or gold implantation was the only method of controlling high-risk proliferative diabetic retinopathy until laser photocoagulation became available. The use of photocoagulation as a treatment in diabetic retinopathy arose from the observation that patients with chorioretinal scarring had less retinopathy. This led early pioneers to use light photocoagulation to generate chorioretinal scars with good results. In the 1940s, Gerd Meyer-Shwickerath, a German ophthalmologist, used sunlight collected from the roof of his hospital and delivered through a system of mirrors to the clinic. Later he developed the xenon light source, which produced sufficiently intense white light to photocoagulate the retina. A relatively large burn subtending between 3° and 8° was produced, and the light intensity was difficult to control. Intense burns penetrate deep into the choroid, causing pain, and in consequence the eyelids had to be held open and ocular anaesthesia was required. The peripheral retina and choroid were often completely ablated following panretinal xenon photocoagulation, and only tubular visual fields remained. The first lasers (Light Amplification by Stimulated Emission of Radiation) were produced in the early 1960s and used for retinal photocoagulation about 3 years later. The extra precision and power provided by lasers proved extremely advantageous, and most photocoagulation today is carried out using laser light of a variety of wavelengths.

How lasers work

Lasers generate electromagnetic radiation which is monochromatic (all the light waves are of the same wavelength) and coherent (all the peaks and troughs of the light waves are in synchrony). Atoms of a gas, such as argon, are contained in a tube with mirrors at each end. The atoms are stimulated to undergo a 'quantum jump' to a higher energy level. When the atom drops back to its original state, it emits light at a particular wavelength related to the energy level. The light bounces up and down the tube, the length of which is an exact multiple of the wavelength. In this way a 'standing wave' is set up, which helps to stimulate more atoms to undergo the energy shift, in a similar way to a standing wave in an organ pipe. At one end of the tube the mirror is half silvered so that light can be 'bled' out of the end. The emitted laser energy can be modified depending upon the type and extent of treatment required.

Lasers are attached to a modified slit lamp biomicroscope, and light is directed into the eye through a contact lens, usually a Goldmann three-mirror lens. Laser photocoagulation can also be performed through a hand-held lens with a special protective coating. In the original lasers, the light beam itself was used to aim the burn. In modern laser systems there is a separate coaxial diode laser for positioning. This provides greater safety for the operator, as it is less likely that small amounts of laser light are reflected back into the ophthalmologist's eye. Modern lasers also have filters in the operator's optics to prevent reflections and flashbacks. The spot size varies from 50 µm up to about 2000 µm either continuously or in discrete steps, depending on the instrument. Most lasers are able to deliver up to 1 W of energy. The energy level is determined by the operator according to the patient's ocular pigmentation and the intensity of burn required. Power is measured in milliwatts and kept as low as possible. The aim is to use the minimum power necessary to produce a threshold burn in the retinal pigment epithelium (RPE). The operator begins at low power (100 mW) and increases the power until 'blanching' of the RPE is seen. With a further increase in power the burn is seen as whitish-grey and then as marble white. Photocoagulation is associated with a rise in temperature to about 30°C, which coagulates proteins, producing a burn. Tissue damage occurs in fractions of a second with high levels of irradiance, but may take several hours at lower levels. Heaping of RPE at the margins of the burn occurs immediately following a high-intensity burn. Heat absorbed by the RPE is dissipated round the burn and transferred to adjacent areas such as the sensory retina and choroid. Photochemical damage therefore occurs in areas adjacent to a visible burn due to both thermal effects and light scatter. The intention is to minimize possible damage to the nerve fibre layer, which might cause an arcuate scotoma (Figure 7.1). Intraocular light scatter is greatest for short wavelengths. Photic damage to short wavelength

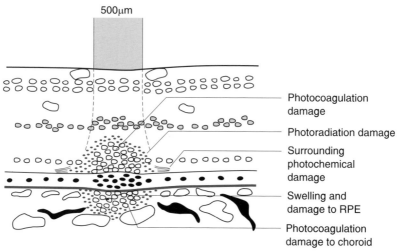

Figure 7.1 Diagrammatic representation of an argon laser burn at 500 μm spot size. This shows the burn centred on the pigment epithelium and the diminishing effect of the heat dissipated on the surrounding structures. Reproduced from Hamilton *et al.*, 1996 by kind permission of the BMJ Publishing Group. © BMJ Publishing Group 1996.

photoreceptors can occur at intensities much less that that required to produce a burn, and scattered light during photocoagulation can result in transient or permanent acquired tritan (blue) colour deficiency.

The argon laser is suitable for most clinical uses, but other lasers that emit different wavelengths may be selected to minimize unwanted absorption or to target specific structures (Table 7.1).

Laser light energy is absorbed by three intraocular pigments; melanin (in the photoreceptors, RPE and choroid), haemoglobin and xanthophyll. Xanthophyll is present in the yellow macular pigment and also in the crystalline lens. Lens pigment density increases with age and in cataract. Unwanted absorption may prevent sufficient light reaching the RPE to produce a therapeutic burn. Macular pigment

Table 7.1 Lasers available for ophthalmic use

Laser	Wavelengths emitted
Argon	488 nm and 514 nm
Dye	577 nm to 630 nm
Krypton	647 nm
Diode	810 nm

pervades the inner and outer plexiform layers, and absorption of laser light is likely to damage these tissues.

Absorption in the RPE is maximal for short wavelengths. Long wavelengths penetrate deeper into the choroid and are more likely to cause pain during photocoagulation treatment. The main peaks of the argon laser are 488 nm (blue) and 514 nm (green). In modern lasers it is possible to remove the blue wavelength with an additional filter so that photocoagulation can be performed with 514 nm only. This reduces intraocular light scatter as well as absorption in the macular pigment. However, only about 40 per cent of laser energy is delivered in the blue wavelength, and both wavelengths are needed if high energy is required. Dye lasers emit several wavelengths. The orange wavelength (577 nm) is absorbed by haemoglobin but not by xanthophyll, and can be used to photocoagulate retinal microaneurysms close to the fovea. Red light produced by the dye laser (630 nm) and by the krypton laser (647 nm) is not absorbed by either haemoglobin or xanthophyll, and is therefore ideal for treatment to the macula and to photocoagulate RPE underneath haemorrhages. However, only about 20 per cent of krypton light is absorbed by the RPE and the remainder penetrates into the choroid. The appearance of a krypton burn therefore differs from that of an argon burn. The semiconductor infrared diode laser (810 nm) is similar to that used in compact disc players, and has potential for treating new vessels growing forward into the vitreous. Only 8 per cent of diode laser light is absorbed by the RPE, but absorption can be enhanced by pre-operative injection of indocyanin green (795 nm). One disadvantage is that the infrared wavelength is absorbed more deeply in the choroid and can make treatment more painful for the patient. Diode lasers are small and portable. It is likely that diode lasers with shorter wavelengths will become available in the near future.

The spot size and the duration of laser exposure are both controlled by the operator. The larger the burn, the greater the spread of photic damage. A spot size of 50–100 µm is used in treatment to the macula, 100–200 µm for focal treatment and a larger spot size of 200–500 µm for panretinal photocoagulation. The duration of exposure is in the range 0.05–0.2 s, and the burn appears larger as the exposure time increases. A longer exposure time increases the risk of the patient's eye moving while the laser is firing, and a shorter time needs more energy to produce the same result.

Accidents with ophthalmic lasers are rare, but they do present a hazard to both the patient and the operator as well as to other personnel. Laser rooms should be designed so that a warning light over the door prevents entry of other personnel when the laser is being used.

Indications for lasers in the treatment of diabetic retinopathy

Photocoagulation may be used for two quite separate reasons in diabetic retinopathy; focal maculopathy or proliferative retinopathy.

Proliferative retinopathy One modality of laser photocoagulation is that of panretinal photocoagulation (PRP), otherwise known as scatter treatment, for the treatment of proliferative retinopathy. Approximately 2000 burns are applied peripherally and within the blood vessel arcades, sparing the central retina round the fovea and up to the optic disc (Figure 7.2). The efficacy of this treatment was the subject of one of the first major randomized controlled clinical trials in ophthalmology, The Diabetic Retinopathy Study Research Group (1976). In this study patients with proliferative retinopathy were treated with 1600 burns to one eye, the other eye acting as a control. After a follow-up period of 2 years, the rate of severe visual loss in the untreated eyes was twice that in the treated eyes.

Full scatter treatment consists of a minimum of 1200 burns, each of 500 µm and 0.05–0.2 s duration. This can usually be achieved in one session using the laser automatic rapid firing function. Burns are placed one spot-size interval apart. Following treatment the patient's vision is likely to be blurred for up to 10 days, possibly longer in Type 2 diabetes. This is thought to be due to temporary macular oedema caused by disruption of the blood retinal barrier. The patient is reassessed 2–4 weeks after treatment. At this time, previously observed disc new vessels (DNV) will have regressed completely in about 50 per cent of patients. When DNV persist, an additional 'fill in' treatment of 1000–1500 burns is given with the burns placed in between the previous laser scars. The patient is reassessed again following a further 2–4 weeks. Some eyes may require still more laser treatment after this period, but treatment is more painful if the burns overlap previous laser scars (Aylward et al., 1989). Peripheral laser scars can be quite large, approximately one-fifth of the disc area, with features of atrophy and hyperpigmentation (Figure 7.2). Panretinal laser scars often become confluent with age, and may cause retinal atrophy and visual field defects. Vitrectomy is considered when photocoagulation is carried out too late to prevent ongoing prolifera- tion resulting in large non-clearing vitreous haemorrhage.

The report of the Early Treatment Diabetic Retinopathy Study Group (1991) suggests that panretinal photocoagulation may benefit some patients with severe non-proliferative retinopathy. The decision whether to treat is based on the features of the retinopathy and the possible

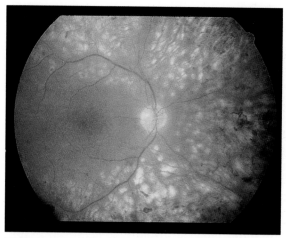

Figure 7.2 Fundus photograph of an eye that has received panretinal photocoagulation. Note sparing of the macular area and some pigment disturbance.

rate of progression to proliferative retinopathy (see Hamilton *et al.*, 1996).

The mode of action of this type of laser treatment is controversial. Laser energy is absorbed by the outer retina and retinal pigment epithelium, but it is the inner retina that is ischaemic. It is probable that the treatment favourably affects the oxygen gradient throughout the retina, thus relieving the ischaemia of the inner retinal layers, and the production of the neovascularizing substance is then reduced, leading to resolution of the new vessels.

New vessels elsewhere (NVE) are treated with laser photocoagulation directed to the area underneath and immediately surrounding them, with possible additional scatter photocoagulation (500–800 burns) to the involved quadrant of the retina.

All diabetic patients with a history of proliferative retinopathy should be carefully screened for recurrent new vessels. These are generally small and have limited growth potential. Treatment is usually with focal photocoagulation.

Maculopathy Laser treatment of diabetic maculopathy has been shown to be effective in preventing visual loss in several large random-ized controlled trials. Its effectiveness depends upon the type of maculopathy and the severity of visual loss. It is most effective in focal maculopathy.

In *focal maculopathy*, the function of the macula is compromised or threatened by abnormalities of the vascular circulation to the macula. There are discrete areas of vascular abnormality causing focal leakage. Lipid is often precipitated at the margin of the abnormal area, resulting in a complete or partial ring of hard exudates. The vascular anomalies responsible are usually microaneurysms, which can be identified by fluorescein angiography. These aneurysms can be targeted for laser photocoagulation, which is generally successful at stopping the leakage, leading to a resolution of oedema and hard exudates. Thus the laser scars are seen as a localized pattern (Figure 7.3).

The blue 488 nm wavelength of the argon laser is contraindicated. A number of longer wavelengths are suitable (Olk, 1990). The spot size is usually 50–100 μm, with an exposure time of 0.05–0.1 s. Minimal power is used to blanch the RPE or microaneurysm. Extensive areas of leakage associated with large circinate rings and multiple leaking sites are treated with a larger spot size, such as 200 μm, and burns are placed in a grid pattern of 100–200 burns spaced at intervals of size corresponding to the diameter of the spot. The laser is focused on the RPE beneath the leaking area. The fovea and parafoveal avascular zone is always avoided. Patients are reassessed about 4 weeks following treatment. Any persistent or additional microaneurysms or areas of leakage are treated if there is a threat to central vision.

This form of maculopathy shows the best response to laser photocoagulation. There is controversy concerning the exact mechanism at work in these cases. Most of the laser energy bypasses the microaneurysm and is absorbed at the level of the retinal pigment epithelium. In addition, the microaneurysms may open again even if they are apparently closed at the time of treatment. It may well be that a general response of the RPE to the laser is responsible for resolution of the oedema, rather than a

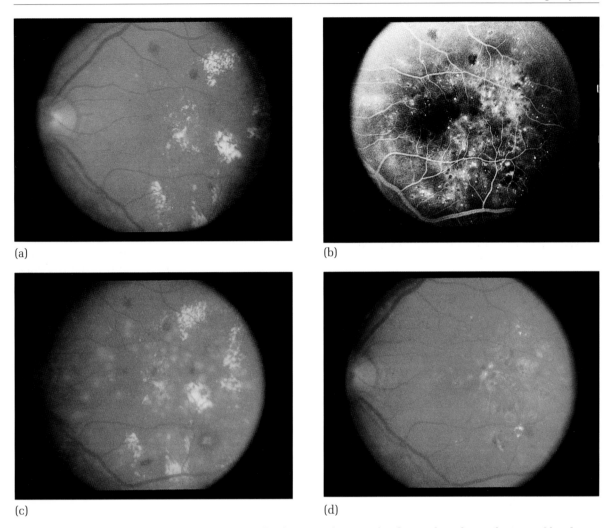

(a)

(b)

(c)

(d)

Figure 7.3 (a) Pre-treatment fundus photograph of an eye showing focal maculopathy with rings of hard exudates associated with focal microaneurysm and other intraretinal microvascular abnormalities. (b) Pre-treatment fluorescein angiogram of the same eye highlighting the leaking microaneurysms. (c) The same eye immediately following focal laser photocoagulation and (d) 3 months later, showing resolution of the maculopathy and positions of the laser burns.

direct effect of the laser on the microaneurysms themselves.

Ischaemic maculopathy is characterized by the closure of capillaries supplying the inner retina at the fovea. The resulting lack of blood supply leads to a permanent dysfunction of the retina, which does not respond to treatment.

Diffuse macular oedema results from generalized leakage of fluid from macular capillaries. This leads to thickening of the retina and reduced function. The application of a grid of light laser burns in the area between the vascular arcades can result in resolution of the oedema, but improvement in visual acuity is rare.

Laser scars after macula treatment are usually small, approximately one-tenth of the disc area, and may appear as round patches of pigment or of atrophy surrounded by pigment. Confluent laser scars are not usually seen after recent macula treatment, although scars can enlarge with time.

Patient set-up

Laser treatment for diabetic retinopathy is usually administered in the outpatient department.

1. Most patients are prepared for treatment by dilating the pupil and applying topical anaesthesia.
2. A contact lens (such as a three- or four-mirror Goldmann type or Panfunduscopic lens) is applied which, along with an adapted slit lamp biomicroscope, allows both visualization and treatment of most of the retina except the far periphery.
3. For PRP, a circular area centred on the fovea and reaching to the disc is usually spared.
4. When applying laser for a PRP, the number of burns that can be applied is very dependent on the co-operation of the patient. Many patients are able to tolerate a full PRP in a single session, though some prefer a number of separate sessions. Some patients feel the laser burns more than others, but if there is excessive discomfort an injection of local anaesthetic (retrobulbar or peribulbar) can be used.
5. For focal treatment, burns can be applied up to one disc diameter from the foveola (depending on how still the patient is!).

Complications of laser treatment

Complications of laser treatment include:

1. Pain – some patients find laser photocoagulation painful. Often the pain increases with subsequent treatments. This may be due to the excessive absorption of laser energy by the pigmented areas from previous treatment sessions. As mentioned above, topical anaesthesia is used routinely to aid application of the fundus contact lens; however, occasionally peribulbar, retrobulbar or even general anaesthesia is required in order to provide adequate treatment.
2. Increasing macular oedema – patients with macula oedema who receive PRP may experience a worsening of their central vision due to an increase in oedema. Usually this is temporary and improves over a few weeks.
3. Visual field defects – PRP can produce a marked loss of visual field, which may be particularly disturbing to the patient at night. In some cases the field may be less than that required by the DVLA for a driving licence. The extent and depth of the visual field loss is dependent on the amount of laser treatment given and the depth of absorption of the laser energy.

There may be other reports of visual loss. Excessive PRP in one session can rarely result in shallowing of the anterior chamber and detachment of the ciliary body, and individual laser burns may damage the fovea or parafoveal retina or induce choroidal neovascularization. Thankfully these complications are very rare. The most common cause of visual loss following laser treatment is the progression of the underlying disease, and many patients will blame the laser treatment for the progression.

Vitrectomy surgery

Vitrectomy is now just over 25 years old. Prior to its invention, the vitreous was considered to be a 'no go' area by ophthalmic surgeons. This ethos stemmed from the serious complications encountered when the vitreous was inadvertently disturbed – for example, rupture of the posterior lens capsule during cataract surgery. Complications such as retinal detachment, cystoid macular oedema and chronic inflammation could ensue. From a surgical aspect, the problem is that the gel structure of vitreous prevents simple aspiration. Any suction that is applied to it results in traction elsewhere, which can result in retinal tears and other problems. If vitreous presented during cataract, a sponge and scissors technique was used to clear it from the wound and anterior segment. A small tongue of gel would be picked up with a cellulose sponge and then divided with scissors.

The first full vitrectomy was carried out by David Kasner in Miami. He used a sponge and scissors technique to remove the vitreous through a very large pars plana incision in an eye with dense amyloid deposits. This procedure was observed by a young researcher at the Bascom Palmer Eye Institute called Robert Machemer. He worked closely with Jean-Marie Parel, a bioengineer, to develop a single device that would suck and cut at the same time. The result of this collaboration was known as the vitreous infusion suction cutter (VISC), and was soon applied to previously inoperable problems such as vitreous opacities.

Further developments of instrumentation followed. Connor O'Mally, working with Steve Charles, introduced the concept of a separate infusion and suction cutter. This allowed smaller diameter instruments to be used, and forms the basis of modern vitrectomy techniques.

Indications for vitrectomy surgery

It is an unfortunate fact that many diabetic patients come to surgery despite the effectiveness of laser in dealing with neovascularization when applied at the appropriate time. Many of these patients are unaware of their proliferative retinopathy until it is quite advanced; hence the need for screening. Surgery is indicated for complications of neovascularization.

Vitreous haemorrhage Vitreous haemorrhage results from bleeding new vessels. The extent of the haemorrhage can vary from a few wisps of vitreous blood to a totally opaque vitreous. Many haemorrhages clear spontaneously, but some do not and require surgical intervention. The time most surgeons wait before intervening depends on a number of factors, but is generally getting shorter. This is because the risks of surgery are getting less as techniques improve and there is an appreciation that the retinopathy continues to progress behind the haemorrhage.

Traction retinal detachment New vessels represent a risk of vitreous haemorrhage, but they can also lead to other more serious problems. As they grow they lay down fibrovascular tissue, which grows along the retinal surface and the posterior vitreous face. The fibrous tissue is prone to contract, producing traction on the retina. Such traction may result in a localized retinal detachment as the retina is tented up by the contracting tissue. If there is traction due to new vessel growth along both vascular arcades then the macula may be tented up between the two areas, producing a 'table-top' macular detachment.

Traction retinal detachments (TRD) tend to be stable and localized, since the majority of the retina remains attached due to the action of the 'RPE pump'. RPE cells actively transport fluid into the choroid, resulting in a negative pressure in the subretinal space. Occasionally continued traction results in the development of a retinal hole, which breaks the suction and leads to a rapid extension of the area of detachment. This configuration is known as a combined rhegmatogenous/traction retinal detachment. Surgical intervention is required if a TRD involves the macula, or if a combined detachment develops.

Surgery for diabetic detachment is much more difficult than surgery for vitreous haemorrhage alone. This is because of the difficulty in relieving the traction caused by the fibrovascular membranes. Such membranes are attached to the underlying retina by vascular 'pegs', and attempts to simply peel the membrane off result either in tearing of these pegs and consequent haemorrhage, or in tearing of the retina. The surgeon must identify the location of the pegs and deal with them in one of two ways. Delamination involves using of horizontally cutting scissors to divide the pegs cleanly and allow the overlying membrane to be released. Segmentation uses vertically cutting scissors to divide the membrane between the pegs, thus relieving the traction between them. In *en bloc* dissection, the initial vitrectomy is deliberately left incomplete so that residual antero-posterior traction can aid the surgeon in identifying the pegs and separating the fibrovascular membrane from the retina.

Once the traction has been relieved, gas or oil may be used to tamponade any breaks that were found or were caused by the surgery. Such breaks can then be sealed with laser. Further laser panretinal photocoagulation is performed if active neovascularization persists.

Surgical techniques for vitrectomy

Three incisions, or ports, are made through the pars plana, between 3.5 and 4.5 mm behind the limbus. One contains a fluid infusion connected to a bag, which replaces the volume of excised tissue and maintains the intraocular pressure. The pressure is determined by the height of the bag above the eye, and is usually set at between 30 and 40 mmHg. A fibre optic 'light pipe' is inserted through one of the other ports, and the remaining one is used to accommodate various instruments. Chief among these is the suction cutter, which is used to remove the vitreous. When this has been done, then a variety of other instruments can be inserted through the same port. These include scissors, forceps, picks and laser probes.

Simple vitrectomy The most common vitrectomy technique for diabetic retinopathy is

vitrectomy and laser. A full pars plana vitrectomy is performed to remove opacified gel. Endolaser photocoagulation is then carried out to reduce the risk of further neovascularization.

Complex vitrectomy If significant fibrovascular traction is present, then the surgery becomes much more complicated. Fibrovascular tissue forms along the surface of the retina and contracts, leading to traction retinal detachment. Often this is associated with a retinal break (combined traction and rhegmatogenous retinal detachment). The main surgical problem is the removal of the fibrovascular tissue with minimal damage to the underlying retina. The sheets of tissue are loosely adherent to the retina except for firm attachments to branches of retinal blood vessels (vascular pegs). These attachments prevent removal of the tissue by simple peeling (as for an epiretinal membrane), as any attempt to peel the fibrous tissue results in tearing of either the retina, producing a hole, or of the vessel, producing a haemorrhage.

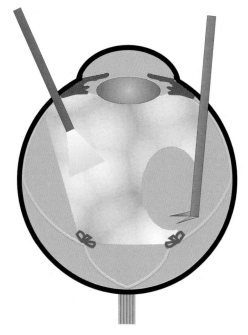

(a)

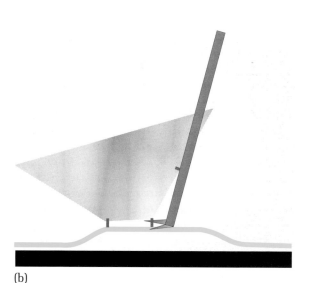

(b)

Figure 7.4 (a) Schematic diagram of a partial vitrectomy performed to allow space to work, and delamination scissors inserted to separate hyaloid from the underlying retina. (b) The tissue is held together by 'small pegs', possibly small blood vessels, which must be identified and cut.

Two techniques have been developed to deal with this problem. Segmentation involves division of the fibrous sheets between pegs using vertically cutting scissors (Figure 7.4a). Delamination involves identifying and cleanly dividing the pegs using horizontally cutting scissors (Figure 7.4b).

Complications of vitrectomy

Like any surgical procedure, vitrectomy is not without complications:

1. At the end of the operation, the vitreous cavity contains clear saline from the infusion bag. Often there is some bleeding from the entry sites into the cavity, so that there is often some degree of vitreous haemorrhage remaining the following day. However, without the structure of the vitreous gel to retain it, this usually clears rapidly over a period of a few weeks.
2. Occasionally retinal tears occur associated with the vitrectomy ports. If these are identified during the operation, they can be treated with cryotherapy and gas injection. However, some develop later and can result in retinal detachment.

3. Delamination often results in iatrogenic retinal holes. These are treated in a similar way to entry site breaks. If there are areas of retinal traction that are unresolved, this can prevent closure of breaks and subsequent retinal detachment.
4. For reasons that are poorly understood, vitrectomy accelerates progression of cataract. If the lens is touched during the procedure, then cataract can develop rapidly.

Other complications include expulsive haemorrhage and infection. These are thankfully rare, probably due to the infusion, which maintains an even intraocular pressure and washes out potential contaminants.

Results of treatments

The results of vitrectomy and laser for simple vitreous haemorrhage are good. There is a very high success rate in terms of removing the opacity and achieving control of the neovascular process. The visual results, however, will depend on the state of the macula, which may be compromised by maculopathy. If the macula is normal, then a successful vitrectomy and

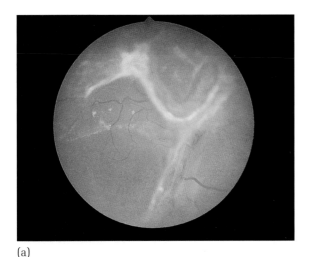

(a)

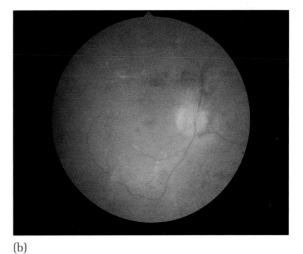

(b)

Figure 7.5 (a) Fundus photograph of the posterior pole of an eye with severe combined traction and rhegmatogenous retinal detachment. (b) The same eye 2 months following successful surgery.

laser would be expected to restore normal vision.

The results of complex vitrectomy are usually less good. The presence of fibrovascular traction means that the incidence of postoperative retinal detachment is higher. In most cases the macular retina is detached preoperatively (see indications) and its function is therefore compromised. In addition, the severity of the neovascularization is associated with macular ischaemia, which can also compromise the visual results. Figure 7.5a shows a fundus photograph of the posterior pole of an eye with severe combined traction and rhegmatogenous retinal detachment. The optic disc and macula are distorted and barely recognizable, and the vision was hand-movements only. Figure 7.5b shows the same eye 2 months following successful surgery; the vision had improved to 6/18.

Future developments

Better control The evidence is very strong that the ocular and other complications of diabetes are directly related to the wide fluctuations in serum glucose associated with diabetes. Therefore it is likely that improvements in the primary treatment of diabetes will have a profound effect on the incidence and severity of diabetic retinopathy. In the absence of such improvements, there are several developments in the field of ophthalmology that are likely to have an impact on diabetic retinopathy.

Screening Current treatment modalities, particularly laser photocoagulation, appear to be extremely effective when delivered early in the course of the disease. Many of the patients who require advanced vitreoretinal surgery may have avoided the need for surgery if their disease had been detected earlier. There is a very good case for a co-ordinated screening programme for diabetic retinopathy, and it is to be hoped that improvements in screening will bring about a reduction in the prevalence of advanced disease.

Pharmacological vitrectomy The vitreous acts like a scaffold for the development of new vessels and fibrovascular traction. Much effort is being directed towards breaking down the gel structure of the vitreous using pharmacological methods. Various enzymes act against elements of the vitreous, such as collagenase and chondroitinase. These agents have had mixed success, and suffer from the non-specific side-effects that are to be expected of any enzymatic agent. Recent work is focusing on the small molecules that bind long collagen fibres together. If such molecules could be blocked by specific inhibitors then the gel structure would collapse with very little chance of unwanted side-effects.

References

Aylward, G. W., Pearson, R. V., Jagger, J. D. and Hamilton, A. M. P. (1989). Extensive argon laser photocoagulation in the treatment of proliferative retinopathy. *Br. J. Ophthalmol.*, **73**, 196–201.

Early Treatment Diabetic Retinopathy Study Group (1991). *Ophthalmology*, **98**(Suppl. 5), 739–834.

Hamilton, A. M. P., Ulbig, M. W. and Polkinghorne, P. (1996). *Management of Diabetic Retinopathy.* BMJ Publishing Group.

Olk, R. J. (1990). Argon green (514 nm) verses krypton red (647 nm) modified grid laser photocoagulation for diffuse diabetic macular oedema. *Ophthalmology*, **97**, 1101–13.

The Diabetes Control and Complications Trial Research Group (1993). The effect of intensive treatment of diabetes on the development and progression of long-term complications in insulin-dependent diabetes mellitus. *N. Engl. J. Med.*, **329**, 977–86.

The Diabetic Retinopathy Study Research Group (1976). Preliminary report of effects of photocoagulation therapy. *Am. J. Ophthalmol.*, **81**, 383–96.

Further reading

British Multicentre Study Group (1983). Photocoagulation for diabetic maculopathy. *Diabetes*, **32**, 1010–16.

Michels, R. G. (1978). Vitrectomy for complications of diabetic retinopathy. *Arch. Ophthalmol.*, **96**, 237–46.

Chapter 8

Visual function in diabetic patients

Jennifer Birch

Introduction

The provision of diabetic care varies in different geographic areas in the United Kingdom. The large numbers of diabetic patients attending medical clinics may preclude routine ophthalmoscopy on all patients at each visit. Although the situation is gradually improving, there is a perceived need for a non-invasive screening test to select patients who would benefit from ophthalmoscopy. A number of examination methods have been studied to find out if the onset of diabetic retinopathy, or progression of retinopathy to a stage needing referral, can be clearly identified (Ishmail and Whitaker, 1998). Ideally the test should be robust, inexpensive, quick and easy to administer. Visual acuity, contrast sensitivity, colour vision, dark adaptation and electrodiagnostic tests have all been considered. This type of screening is challenging because most diabetic patients are over 50 years of age due to the high prevalence of Type 2 disease. Small pupil size and increased lens density are confounding factors. Comparison of results obtained by diabetic patients and age-matched controls may be inadequate because age-related changes occur at an earlier age in diabetes. In many cases it would be more appropriate to match visual function in diabetic patients with normal subjects at least 10 years older. Individual studies have examined different patient cohorts, and it is not unexpected that results differ in detail and that test efficiency (sensitivity and specificity) is found to vary. Although

some studies reach statistical significance, the results generally fail to achieve clinical relevance. For example, although the difference between the mean values for diabetic and non-diabetic patients may be statistically significant, it may be impossible to categorize individual patients because the standard deviations are too large. As yet, no visual function test fulfils the desired aims. The present emphasis in diabetes care is therefore to deliver ophthalmoscopy in the most cost-effective way. It is this policy that has involved more optometrists in co-management of diabetic patients.

Visual function in diabetic retinopathy

Subtle visual function deficits have been found in some diabetic patients prior to the onset of ophthalmoscopically visible retinopathy. This has led to a debate as to whether these are due to poor diabetic control at the time of the examination, undetected retinal microvascular abnormalities deep in the capillary bed (not shown in fluorescein angiograms) or subclinical neurological disease (North et al., 1997). In most cases, changes in visual function correlate with the features of retinopathy. Visual function is within normal limits or minimally affected in background retinopathy, compromised in proliferative retinopathy and profoundly affected in maculopathy.

Laser photocoagulation aims to preserve visual acuity, but can produce other changes in visual function (Cambie, 1980). The severity of these changes depends on the pre-treatment status of the patient, the type and amount of treatment and any post-treatment complications.

Visual acuity and contrast sensitivity

Most diabetic patients with background retinopathy have normal visual acuity of 6/6 or better (Kohner *et al.*, 1998). However, careful measurement of Snellen visual acuity, when the patient is examined in the same office at each visit, may show a slight but significant worsening (by one or two lines) with increased severity of retinopathy. Visual acuity can be within normal limits in severe pre-proliferative and proliferative retinopathy unless macular traction is present. Visual acuity is therefore a poor guide to the development of sight-threatening retinopathy. Significantly reduced visual acuity is associated with maculopathy, particularly macular oedema (Bresnick *et al.*, 1985). There is sudden dramatic loss of vision following vitreous haemorrhage.

Contrast sensitivity has been measured with grating patterns on an oscilloscope and with photographic plates. The usefulness of contrast sensitivity as a screening tool to identify the onset of retinopathy (or the developing features of retinopathy) remains a matter of debate, but most tests produce an unacceptably high number of false positive results, especially in patients over 50 years of age (Ghafour *et al.*, 1982). Contrast sensitivity is reduced for all spatial frequencies in diabetic maculopathy in step with reduction in Snellen visual acuity.

Visual fields and dark adaptation

Assessment of peripheral visual fields is not a realistic option for identifying diabetic retinopathy. Transient relative scotomas occur over areas of poorly perfused retina. In proliferative retinopathy, absolute scotomas are found distal to the point of peripheral neovascularization and over clusters of abnormal features (Greite *et al.*, 1981). Abnormalities in the central visual field can be demonstrated with Amsler charts in maculopathy.

Panretinal photocoagulation can produce both absolute and relative scotomas in the peripheral field, which may be noticed by the patient. The earliest panretinal treatment regimes with the xenon arc or long duration argon burns produced permanent 'tubular' fields (Zingirian *et al.*, 1977). Modern treatment styles, using the filtered argon (green) laser and short duration burns, aim to preserve the inner nuclear layer and minimize field loss. Field loss therefore depends on the intensity and depth of the burn and on the amount of treatment. Paracentral scotomas are produced by grid laser photocoagulation. The extent of field loss may increase slightly with time although no further treatment is given.

Final dark adaptation thresholds for diabetic patients without retinopathy are greater than normal values for the person's age (Henson and North, 1979). However, dark adaptation is within normal limits if the smaller pupil size is taken into account. Poor night vision is a symptom of pre-proliferative and proliferative diabetic retinopathy, and occurs as a consequence of poor mesopic and scotopic pupil dilation as well as extensive scotomas in the peripheral field. All patients with proliferative retinopathy have elevated final rod thresholds, which correlate with the extent of peripheral retinal ischemia. Elevation of the final rod threshold corresponds with the extent of peripheral field loss following panretinal photocoagulation (Cambie, 1980).

Small pupil size, loss of peripheral visual field and poor dark adaptation may affect the ability to drive, especially at night.

Electrodiagnostic tests

Electrodiagnostic procedures require dedicated equipment and examiner expertise. The tests themselves need only take a few minutes. Pattern electroretinograms (PERG) have the potential for identifying the stage of retinopathy when referral is required. Values are within normal limits in background retinopathy and are reduced below the normal value at the pre-proliferative stage, when 'cotton wool spots' and areas of capillary non-perfusion are present (Arden *et al.*, 1986). In some measurement conditions, small wavelets known as oscillatory potentials can be demonstrated on the ascending limb of the b wave. These wavelets are specifically related to vascular integrity. Oscillatory potentials decrease in amplitude in background retinopathy and are absent in proliferative retinopathy. However, measurement of oscillatory potentials is too variable to use as a screening test for proliferative retinopathy. In proliferative retinopathy both the photopic and scotopic b waves decrease in amplitude and there is a delay in response time.

Colour vision

Acquired Type 3 (tritan) colour deficiency was first described in diabetic patients with retinopathy by Dubois-Poulsen and Cochet in 1954, and a large number of papers on acquired colour deficiency in diabetes have been published since that date. Subtle losses of hue discrimination ability for desaturated colours and increases in the matching range for tritan metameric matches have been reported prior to the onset of visible retinopathy (Banford *et al.*, 1994; Kurtenbach *et al.*, 1999). This is associated with reduced sensitivity in the short wavelength (S or blue cone) visual pathway measured psychophysically (Greenstein *et al.*, 1990). Identification of acquired tritan colour deficiency could therefore potentially detect diabetic retinopathy. However, screening tests for tritan deficits have low sensitivity and specificity due to individual variations in pre-retinal absorption by macular pigment and lens density.

Results obtained from colour vision test batteries show that the severity of acquired colour deficiency correlates with the features of the retinopathy and the extent of field loss (Birch *et al.*, 1980). Both clinical and psychophysical tests show that the acquired defect passes through a number of stages that are typical of Type 3 colour deficiency (Birch, 1998). Initially there is specific loss of short wavelength (blue) sensitivity and typical tritan responses are made on pseudoisochromatic and hue discrimination tests. In later stages the long wavelength (red) and middle wavelength (green) mechanisms are involved, and there is an abnormal response to the Ishihara plates and poor overall hue discrimination is found with the Farnsworth-Munsell 100 hue test. Acquired tritanopia may occur in both the initial and late stages. Colour vision is particularly poor in diabetic maculopathy, even when visual acuity is relatively good (6/18) (Bresnick *et al.*, 1985). Congenital red-green dichromats may have almost complete absence of colour discrimination when an acquired Type 3 (tritan) deficiency develops.

Both congenital colour deficiency and severe acquired colour deficiency can adversely affect the patient's ability to perform self urine analysis using colour coded materials (Bresnick *et al.*, 1984) and poor diabetic control can result (Thompson *et al.*, 1979). An abnormal result with the Ishihara plates indicates that colour coded methods for monitoring diabetic control should either be undertaken by another family member or substituted for another which provides information on a digital display. Acquired colour deficiency may impact on the patient's work and lifestyle. It may not be possible to continue in an occupation that requires normal colour vision.

Changes in colour vision following panretinal photocoagulation are due to the effect of intense prolonged light scatter in the optic media during treatment and to loss of receptor fields caused by the burns themselves. Retinal receptors are most susceptible to damage by short wavelength light. This can occur at much lower intensities than required to produce a therapeutic burn. The argon laser emits strongly in two wavelengths, 488 nm and 513 nm. Most retinal damage is caused by the shorter wavelength, and this is now routinely filtered during photocoagulation. Older style argon laser panretinal photocoagulation, using both wavelengths and long exposure times, produced permanent Type 3 colour deficiency, often acquired tritanopia (Birch and Hamilton, 1981). Patients treated with central grid photocoagulation usually have very poor colour vision.

Transient colour vision changes may be noticed by the patient immediately following modern panretinal photocoagulation treatment with short duration filtered argon (green) laser burns. This may be due to temporary damage caused by light scatter during treatment or to post-operative macular oedema. Full recovery takes place within 1–2 weeks.

Changes in visual function due to abnormalities in the anterior eye

Cataract Cataract is an important cause of visual loss in diabetic patients (see Chapter 5). Age-related cataract occurs at a younger age than in the normal population, and women in the 50–64 years age group are particularly at risk. Diabetic patients benefit from early cataract extraction if visual symptoms are present or if visualization of the fundus, to identify retinal thickening, is impeded. Significant cataract may prevent effective photocoagulation treatment. Diabetic patients should therefore be referred to an ophthalmologist at an earlier stage than non-diabetic patients.

Glaucoma A higher prevalence of chronic open angle glaucoma has been reported in diabetes, but this may be due to a higher detection rate than in the general population because patients are under ophthalmological supervision. The use of pilocarpine is contraindicated because the small pupil size prevents a good view of the retina. Diabetic lenses are larger than average for the patient's age, and this carries an increased risk of primary angle closed glaucoma (see Chapter 5).

Refractive error Poor metabolic control may result in rapid fluctuations in refractive error, possibly due to refractive index changes in the lens cortex driven by cyclic osmotic hydration and dehydration (Gwinip and Villarreal, 1976). The overall trend is usually towards increased myopia, although hypermetropia has been reported in hyperglycaemic episodes (Eva et al., 1982). About 50 per cent of people who

develop progressive myopia in middle life are found to have Type 2 diabetes. Diet regulation aims to achieve the person's ideal weight gradually over perhaps 6–10 weeks (Chapter 1). Refractive error may change during this period, and it is best to delay a spectacle prescription until good control, with stable body weight, is achieved (Saito et al., 1993). Inexpensive spectacles or 'clip on' lenses can be considered as an interim measure. Accommodation may be reduced following panretinal photocoagulation if the long ciliary nerves are damaged.

Corneal sensitivity Loss of corneal sensitivity in diabetic patients is part of generalized sensory neuropathy. Corneal sensitivity is usually within normal limits in patients without retinopathy. Thereafter, reduced sensitivity correlates with the severity of retinopathy and is markedly reduced in proliferative retinopathy (Rogell, 1980; Ruben, 1994). Diabetic patients have an increased risk of keratitis and recurrent corneal erosions. Contact lens wearers need careful supervision.

The iris and pupil The iris may become more bulky due to infiltration with glycogen, and pupil responses are reduced due to peripheral neuropathy. As a result, the diabetic pupil is smaller than average in all age groups and dilates poorly in darkness. Both direct and indirect pupil reflexes are slow and reduced in amplitude (Smith and Smith, 1983). There is also a 'supersensitive' mydriatic response to topical sympathomimetic drugs in excess of the normal age-related response. Good mydriasis may be obtained with a weak solution (2.5%) of phenylephrine unless use of a sympathomimetic drug is contraindicated (Huber et al., 1985). Rubeosis (new blood vessel growth in the iris) is associated with untreated or aggressive proliferative retinopathy, and brings the risk of hyphaema. Neovascularization usually begins at the pupil margin, but in advanced stages a fibrovascular membrane may grow across the trabecular meshwork causing secondary glaucoma.

References

Arden, G. B., Hamilton, A. M., Wilson-Holt, J. *et al.* (1986). Pattern electroretinograms become abnormal when background retinopathy deteriorates to a proliferative stage. Possible use of a screening test. *Br. J. Ophthalmol.*, **70**, 330–35.

Banford, D., North, R. V., Dolben, J. *et al.* (1994). Longitudinal study of visual function in young insulin dependent diabetics. *Ophthal. Physiol. Opt.*, **14**, 339–46.

Birch, J. (1998). *Diagnosis of Colour Deficiency.* Butterworth-Heinemann.

Birch, J. and Hamilton, A. M. (1981). Xenon arc and argon laser photocoagulation in the treatment of disc new vessels: Effect on colour vision. *Trans. Ophthal. Soc. UK*, **101**, 94–8.

Birch, J., Hamilton, A. M. P. and Gould, E. S. (1980). Colour vision in relation to clinical features and extent of field loss in diabetic retinopathy. In: *Colour Deficiencies V* (G. Verriest, ed). Adam Hilger, pp. 83–88.

Bresnick, C. H., Groo, A. and Korth, K. (1984). Urinary glucose testing inaccuracies among diabetic patients. *Arch. Ophthalmol.*, **102**, 1489–96.

Bresnick, G. H., Condit, R. S., Palta, M. *et al.* (1985). Association of hue discrimination loss and diabetic retinopathy. *Arch. Ophthalmol.*, **103**, 1317–24.

Cambie, E. (1980). Functional results following argon laser photocoagulation in eyes with diabetic retinopathy. In: *Diabetic Renal–Retinal Syndrome* (E. A. Friedman and F. A. L'Esperance, eds), pp. 295–307. Crune and Stratton.

Dubois-Poulsen, A. and Cochet, P. (1954). Un cas de dyschromatopsie diabetique. *Bull. Soc. Ophthalmol.* (Paris), **4**, 323–30.

Eva, P. R., Pascoe, P. T. and Vaughan, D. G. (1982). Refractive changes in hyperglycaemia. *Br. J. Ophthalmol.*, **66**, 500–505.

Ghafour, I. M., Foulds, W. S., Allan, D. and McClure, E. (1982). Contrast sensitivity in diabetic patients with and without retinopathy. *Br. J. Ophthalmol.*, **66**, 492–5.

Greite, J. H., Zumbansen, H. P. and Adamczyk, R. (1981). Visual fields in diabetic retinopathy. *Doc. Ophthalmol. Proc. Series* 26, pp. 25–32.

Greenstein, V. C., Sarter, B., Hood, D. *et al.* (1990). Hue discrimination and S cone pathway sensitivity in early diabetic retinopathy. *Invest. Ophthalmol. Vis. Sci.*, **31**, 1732–7.

Gwinup, G. and Villarreal, A. (1976). Relation of serum glucose concentration to changes in refraction. *Diabetes*, **25**, 29–31.

Henson, D. B. and North, R. V. (1979). Dark adaptation in diabetes mellitus. *Br. J. Ophthalmol.*, **63**, 539–41.

Huber, M. J. E., Smith, S. A. and Smith, S. E. (1985). Mydriatic drugs for diabetes. *Br. J. Ophthalmol.*, **69**, 425–7.

Ishmail, G. M. and Whitaker, D. (1998). Early detection of changes in visual function in diabetes mellitus. *Ophthal. Physiol. Opt.*, **18**, 3–12.

Kohner, E. M., Aldington, S. J., Stratton, I. M. *et al.* (1998). United Kingdom Prospective Diabetes Study. *Arch. Ophthalmol.*, **116**, 297–303.

Kurtenbach, A., Scheifer, A. N. and Zrenner, E. (1999). Pre-retinopic changes in colour vision of juvenile diabetics. *Br. J. Ophthalmol.*, **83**, 43–6.

North, R. V., Cooney, O., Chambers, D. *et al.* (1997). Does hyperglycaemia have an influence upon colour vision of patients with diabetes mellitus? *Ophthal. Physiol Opt.*, **17**, 95–101.

Rogell, G. D. (1980). Corneal hyperthesia and retinopathy in diabetes mellitus. *Ophthalmology*, **87**, 229–33.

Ruben, S. T. (1994). Corneal sensation in insulin dependent and non-insulin dependent diabetics with proliferative retinopathy. *Acta Ophthalmol.*, **72**, 576–80.

Saito, Y., Kinoshito, S., Nakamura, K. *et al.* (1993). Transient hyperopia and lens swelling in initial therapy in diabetes. *Br. J. Ophthalmol.*, **77**, 145–8.

Smith, S. A. and Smith, S. E. (1983). The diabetic pupil. *Br. J. Ophthalmol.*, **67**, 89–93.

Thompson, D. G., Howarth, F., Taylor, H. *et al.* (1979). Defective colour vision in diabetes : a hazard to management. *Br. Med. J.*, **1**, 859–60.

Zingirian, M., Pisano, E. and Gandolfo, E. (1977). Visual field damage after photocoagulation treatment for diabetic retinopathy. *Doc. Ophthalmol. Proc. Series 14*, pp. 265–73.

Chapter 9

Screening for diabetic retinopathy
Richard Newsom

Introduction

Screening for diabetic retinopathy is accepted as good clinical practice and cost-effective healthcare (Kohner and Porta, 1991a; Harding *et al.*, 1995; Burns-Cox, 1996; Javitt and Aiello, 1996). The importance of screening for this condition was recognized following the development of effective laser treatment in the 1980s. The Diabetic Retinopathy Study (DRS) showed that panretinal photocoagulation prevented severe visual loss in 50 per cent of patients with 'high risk' proliferative diabetic retinopathy (DRS, 1981), and the Early Treatment Diabetic Retinopathy Study (ETDRS, 1985) showed that visual loss was prevented in 50–70 per cent of patients with exudatative maculopathy.

As visual loss occurs in relatively young patients, it was soon obvious that the cost of blindness in these patients outweighed the cost of screening for diabetic retinopathy in patients with Type 1 and Type 2 diabetes (Javitt and Aiello, 1996). As duration of the disease is a major risk factor for development of retinopathy, more people are likely to develop diabetic eye problems as they live longer with their disease. The risk of diabetes-related visual impairment could be reduced by implementing programmes that detect and treat diabetic retinopathy.

At present it is not clear which is the best method for screening for this condition. Many approaches have been used, and these will be discussed later in the chapter. The Department of Health will shortly be publishing UK guidelines for diabetic retinopathy screening. The British Diabetic Association already has referral guidelines in place, which are similar to those described in Chapter 6. Guidelines may vary, but it is essential, as with other screening programmes in healthcare, that quality control is central; without this any service will be liable to failure and litigation.

Principles of screening

Definition and purpose of screening

Screening involves identifying unrecognized disease or risk factors for disease by applying tests on a large scale to a population that has no symptoms. Screening tests may not be diagnostic in themselves, and usually seek to identify groups at high risk of the condition. Further tests are needed to confirm the diagnosis.

The purpose of screening is to select those people who are at higher risk of developing a disease and to offer them a health intervention aimed at prevention by one of two means:

1. Prevention of serious outcomes of existing disease, e.g. blindness in a diagnosed diabetic patient
2. Prevention of the development of a disease, e.g. screening for high cholesterol levels to

select people at higher risk of coronary heart disease for a health promotion or cholesterol-lowering drug treatment.

This is in contrast to 'case finding' or the diagnosis of disease in self-presenting patients. For example, individuals presenting for an eye examination are usually not representative of a disease spectrum, due to the 'volunteer effect'. They are more aware of their health, seek regular consultations, and are healthier than those who do not present for examination.

Screening may be applied to the whole population (mass screening) or to a selected group with an increased prevalence of a condition (target screening). A target population should be clearly definable in terms of age, sex, occupation or illness, and a screening programme should examine everyone within the population.

For screening to be effective, the disease should fulfil certain criteria. There are WHO guidelines (Wilson and Junger, 1968), which are briefly summarized below:

- the condition screened for should be an important public health problem
- the natural history should be well understood
- there should be a detectable early stage
- there should be benefit from early diagnosis and treatment
- the screening test should be safe and acceptable
- there should be adequate provision for the extra clinical workload resulting from screening
- the costs should be balanced against the benefits.

Well-recognized screening tests are necessary, and these should also fulfil certain criteria. They should be sensitive enough to detect the disease and specific enough to exclude a non-affected individual. As the test will be performed many thousands of times, it should be easy to administer and cause no physical or psychological damage. The test should be widely available to all individuals at risk within the population, and inexpensive. Good administration and clear referral pathways are necessary, as well as audit of the screening test and the patient referral systems.

Assessment of screening tests

Screening tests should be compared to a 'gold standard' to measure their accuracy of case detection. Diseased individuals within a population may be described as 'true positive' (A + C), and those without the disease as 'true negative' (D + B) (Table 9.1).

The screening test aims to distinguish the true positives from the true negatives; however, it may wrongly classify some patients. From Table 9.1, several parameters may be described.

The *sensitivity* is the proportion of affected individuals correctly identified by the screening test. A low sensitivity indicates that many affected individuals have been missed, and have actually tested negative (false negatives).

Sensitivity = $A/(A+C)$
False negative rate = $1 -$ sensitivity

The *specificity* is the proportion of unaffected individuals correctly identified by the screening test. A low specificity indicates a high proportion of unaffected individuals actually tested positive (false positive).

Specificity = $D/(D+B)$
False positive rate = $1 -$ specificity

Table 9.1 Results of a screening test

Result of screening test	True disease status	
	affected	unaffected
positive	A	B
negative	C	D

The *positive predictive value* (PPV) is the odds that a patient with a positive test result has the disease.

$$PPV = A/(A + B)$$

The *negative predictive value* (NPV) is a measure of the probability of the patient truly not having the condition if the screening test result is negative.

$$NPV = D/(C + D)$$

The *odds of being affected given a positive result* (OAPR) is the ratio of the number affected to unaffected individuals among those with a positive screen test result (A : B).

Other demographic data may be described:

Target population	$A + B + C + D$
The test yield	$A/(A + B + C + D)$
The disease prevalence	$(A + C)/(A + B + C + D)$
Screen positive rate	$(A + B)/(A + B + C + D)$

A worked example is shown below:

Target population	$160 + 1 + 40 + 99$	$= 300\ (100\%)$
Prevalence	$= (160 + 40)/(300)$	$= 0.66\ (66\%)$
Sensitivity	$= 160/200$	$= 0.8\ (80\%)$
False negative rate	$= 40/200$	$= 0.2\ (20\%)$
Specificity	$= 99/100$	$= 0.99\ (99\%)$
False positive rate	$= 1/100$	$= 0.01\ (1\%)$
PPV	$= 160/161$	$= 0.99\ (99\%)$
NPV	$= 99/139$	$= 0.71\ (71\%)$
Screen positive rate	$= 161/300$	$= 0.54\ (54\%)$

Most screening tests a strike a balance between a high detection rate and low false positive rate. Increasing the sensitivity (detection rate) increases the yield, but will tend to increase the costs (e.g. of treating more false positive patients and increasing test costs). Using these data a screening test may be evaluated for its usefulness in detecting disease; however, it is equally important to test the screening process as a whole and not just the test itself.

Evaluation of a screening programme

Outcome measures The 'screening process' may be assessed in the same way as a screening test. The number of screened patients appropriately referred for treatment indicates the true positives of the process; those inappropriately referred indicate the false positives. Patients with the disease presenting for treatment and who have not arrived through the screening programme give an indication of false negatives. These may have either not been found by the test or not been selected for screening.

Table 9.2 Results of a screening test: hypothetical example

Result of screening test	True disease status		
	affected	unaffected	total
positive	160	1	161
negative	40	99	139
total	200	100	300

Prevalence and incidence rates for the disease can be determined and give an indication of the expected burden of the disease within a given community, and these may also be a useful guideline as to whether screening is effective or necessary. The proportion of patients referred from different geographical areas may vary with the screening protocol used, and may be a general indicator of the effectiveness of techniques, particularly if there is a disparity between adjacent populations. Similarly, trends in the number of patients treated may vary over time. If there is a sudden increase or decrease in referrals there may be some problem with the screening technique or the referral administration. Referrals should be appropriate and consistent.

Cost-effectiveness Cost-effectiveness is key to a successful screening programme, and the cost of screening and treatment of early disease against that of treatment of late detected disease needs to be evaluated. Costs of screening also include further diagnostic tests as well as the cost of treatment. On the other hand, in the absence of screening, higher costs will be incurred by treatment of patients with more advanced disease. Human and economic costs should also be taken into consideration. The balance of these costs determines whether screening for the disease is viable.

Screening for diabetic retinopathy

Diabetic retinopathy fulfils the criteria for screening. It occurs in a definable population of patients (available from diabetic clinic and general practitioner databases) and is a significant public heath problem, considering there are between 1.2 and 2 million people with diabetes in the UK.

The DRS showed that in eyes with high risk neovascularization, panretinal photocoagulation reduced the risk of severe visual loss from 26 per cent to 11 per cent (DRS, 1978). Similarly, the ETDRS showed that macular photocoagulation reduced the risk of visual loss from diabetic maculopathy by 50 per cent

(ETDRS, 1985). The natural history of diabetic retinopathy is well researched and there is effective treatment; this asymptomatic disease clearly merits screening. Other studies have also shown screening to be effective in reducing the incidence of blindness from diabetic retinopathy (Javitt *et al.*, 1994; Kristinsson *et al.*, 1995). Screening has also been shown to be cost-effective, as the costs of blindness are high, as are the costs of treatment in more advanced stages of the diseases such as vitrectomy (Javitt *et al.*, 1994). There are now several effective screening tests that cause no physical harm and are well-tolerated by patients. However, the provision of screening programmes is not uniform or co-ordinated through the UK.

UK studies have shown that, during an initial screening, 6–9 per cent of patients have sight-threatening retinopathy (proliferative diabetic retinopathy or diabetic maculopathy) (O'Hare *et al.*, 1996); during subsequent rounds this falls to 2 per cent. Similar studies in the USA found 20 per cent of patients with Type 1 diabetes had proliferative disease at baseline screening, and 13 per cent had maculopathy (Klein *et al.*, 1989). In patients with older onset diabetes, proliferative retinopathy was found in 2 per cent of cases and macular oedema in 4 per cent (Klein *et al.*, 1990).

The British Diabetic Association (1994) and the Royal College of Ophthalmologists both emphasize the need for regular audit of a planned screening programme. Indeed, recent public concern over cervical screening programmes has demonstrated the importance of this issue. It is difficult for clinicians to submit to regular review. However, without these safeguards no screening programme will withstand public scrutiny (Harris *et al.*, 1994). The British Diabetic Association (1994) suggests that screening tests for diabetic retinopathy should have a sensitivity of at least 80 per cent; a specificity of at least 95 per cent; a technical failure rate of no more than 5 per cent; and that 0.5–1 per cent of patients should be re-examined using a 'gold standard' technique each year to maintain quality control. The sensitivity and specificity of the whole process should also be regularly checked. Outcomes of referrals to ophthalmology clinics should be recorded and the incidence of diabetic retinopathy. Visual impairment and blindness should be monitored. The organization of the screening process should be carefully analysed, and feedback loops put in place before the screening is started.

Screening for diabetic retinopathy is now well established as good cost-effective healthcare. The disease fits well into the WHO guidelines for screening, having an effective treatment and a well established natural history. What is less certain is the means by which the disease is screened; however, regular audit of both the test (and or tester) and the referral mechanism is essential if visual loss is to be prevented in this condition.

Guidelines for screening for diabetic retinopathy

Two published guidelines for screening for diabetic retinopathy are summarized below.

The St Vincent Declaration Working Group
The St Vincent Declaration Working Group (Kohner and Porta, 1991b) have produced guidelines for screening for the disease. They suggest the aims of screening are three-fold:

- diagnosis of sight-threatening retinopathy requiring treatment
- detection of mild diabetic retinopathy needing follow-up but no treatment
- diagnosis of concomitant eye disease such as cataract or glaucoma.

The American Academy of Ophthalmology, American Congress of Physicians, American Diabetic Association
The American Academy of Ophthalmology, American Congress of Physicians and American Diabetic Association (1992) have also published guidelines for screening for diabetic retinopathy:

- Type 1 patients should be screened for diabetic retinopathy 5 years following diagnosis of diabetes (not indicated before puberty) and annually thereafter

- Type 2 patients should be examined at the time of diagnosis, then

  if diabetic retinopathy is present, yearly
  if diabetic retinopathy is not present, two-yearly until diabetic retinopathy is detected and then annually

- pregnant women should receive pregnancy counselling and be examined pre-pregnancy and then during each trimester of pregnancy (see Chapter 2)
- patients with macular oedema, proliferative, pre-proliferative or severe background diabetic retinopathy should be referred to an eye clinic.

The reader should refer to Chapter 6 for referral criteria for diabetic retinopathy recommended in this book.

Methods used for diabetic retinopathy screening

Introduction Several alternative methods have been proposed for screening for diabetic retinopathy: direct ophthalmoscopy; various methods of fundus photography (see Chapter 10); indirect ophthalmoscopy; indirect ophthalmoscopy using slit lamp biomicroscopy; and fluorescein angiography. Methods may be divided into clinical (direct and indirect ophthalmoscopy, slit lamp biomicroscopy) or photographic (mydriatic, non-mydriatic, Polaroid cameras, digital imaging) methods.

In the literature, different gold standards or reference standards have been used to evaluate the accuracy of a variety of screening test procedures. The gold standard for diabetic retinopathy is seven-field stereo colour fundus photography followed by assessment by a fully trained diabetic retinopathy grader (Moss *et al.*, 1989). This method of grading is time consuming and costly, and other reference standards have been used to evaluate screening tests. These include clinical examination by ophthalmologists or retinal specialists, but unfortunately clinicians also vary in their ability to detect diabetic retinopathy (Mitchell and Moffitt, 1990; Harding *et al.*, 1995). It is difficult to compare studies that use different reference standards as well as different methods of assessment (Newsom, 1991). This chapter discusses the most important findings from some of these studies.

However, direct ophthalmoscopy and non-mydriatic fundus photography appear to be unsatisfactory, and a large proportion of sight-threatening retinopathy can be missed (Moss *et al.*, 1985; Williams *et al.*, 1986; Buxton *et al.*, 1991).

Direct ophthalmoscopy The direct ophthalmoscope has been widely used to detect retinopathy, as it is the most common instrument for retinal examination. Direct ophthalmoscopes provide good magnification and have the advantage of being portable and inexpensive. However, the field of view is limited (about 8°) unless the pupil is dilated. View of the retinal periphery is usually poor, and there is no stereopsis. Screening accuracy is highly operator-dependent, and the technique leaves no objective or permanent record. Sussman *et al.* (1982) showed that relatively experienced clinicians still have difficulty producing reliable results. In this study the reference standard was the consensus of diagnosis of three retinal specialists reviewing seven-field stereo colour fundus photographs (7SFP) and fundus fluorescein angiograms (FFA). They had also performed indirect ophthalmoscopy on the same patients a week previously.

The possible diagnoses were: normal; background retinopathy; diabetic maculopathy; pre-proliferative retinopathy; proliferative retinopathy; or other. Internists, senior medical residents and diabetologists had correct diagnostic rates of 27 per cent, 31 per cent and 36 per cent respectively. General ophthalmologists and retinal specialists had correct diagnostic rates of 52 per cent and 70 per cent respectively (Table 9.3).

Similar findings have been reported by other investigators. Forrest *et al.* (1987) looked at the ability of a diabetologist and a clinical nurse specialist in detecting diabetic retinopathy. Both had a detection rate of about 50 per cent for background diabetic retinopathy compared with fundus photography. The doctor missed proliferative retinopathy 84 per cent of the time, and the nurse missed it 100 per cent of the time. Klein *et al.* (1985a) reported a sensitivity of 50 per cent for proliferative diabetic retinopathy and 51 per cent for background diabetic retinopathy, obtained by an experienced ophthalmic technician examining through undilated pupils, compared with three 30° stereoscopic fundus photographs. Similarly, Kinyoun *et al.* (1992) found that a retinal specialist, using both direct and indirect ophthalmoscopy with dilated pupils, missed approximately 50 per cent of eyes with microaneurysms compared with seven-field stereo photography. Moss *et al.* (1985) found that training and observation through dilated pupils could improve detection rates by up to 86 per cent. Harding *et al.* (1995) reported that direct ophthalmoscopy with dilated pupils, by an experienced ophthalmologist, yielded sensitivity of only 65 per cent for sight-threatening diabetic eye disease compared with a retinal specialist performing slit lamp biomicroscopy.

Table 9.3 Summary of results from Sussman *et al.* (1982)

Clinician	Instrument used	Sensitivity for grading BDR (%)
Internists	Direct ophthalmoscope	48
Senior medical residents	Direct ophthalmoscope	50
Diabetologists	Direct ophthalmoscope	67
General ophthalmologists	Indirect + direct	91
Retinal specialist	Indirect + photo + FFA	100

Macular oedema is unlikely to be reliably detected using this technique because there is no stereopsis.

Indirect ophthalmoscopy using a 20 dioptre (20D) lens Indirect ophthalmoscopy images the retina using a headset and a hand-held lens. The technique offers a large field of view (approximately 60° with a 20D lens), but low magnification (approximately 3×). Moss *et al.* (1985) and Kinyoun *et al.* (1992) reported 86 per cent agreement between direct ophthalmoscopy through dilated pupils, supplemented by indirect ophthalmoscopy when required, compared with seven-field stereophotographs assessed by a trained grader.

Indirect ophthalmoscopy has been superseded by biomicroscopy as the screening method of choice.

Slit lamp binocular indirect ophthalmoscopy
The development of non-contact (hand-held) lenses for use with the slit lamp biomicroscope has revolutionized the examination of the fundus. This technique gives a three-dimensional view of the retina with good magnification, and is the preferred method for diabetic retinopathy screening. Clinical decisions with respect to patient management are most commonly made using this form of retinal examination. Some studies have used slit lamp binocular indirect ophthalmoscopy (BIO) as a reference standard for other methods of screening (Harding *et al.*, 1995). However, diagnosis is open to clinical interpretation, and this leads to variability both within and between studies.

Hammond *et al.* (1996) compared the performance of an optometrist with an ophthalmologist, both using a combination of slit lamp BIO and direct ophthalmoscopy. They found a sensitivity of 92 per cent for sight-threatening background retinopathy and 77 per cent for sight-threatening maculopathy, with an overall sensitivity of 77 per cent. A recent study using hospital-based optometrists using slit lamp BIO compared favourably with an ophalmologist using the same method of examination in 103 patients (Leese *et al.*, 1997). They reported that five of the 92 patients referred for suspected

intraretinal microvascular abnormality or new vessels had no pathology (false positive rate of 5.5 per cent), and one case of macular oedema was not referred (sensitivity 10/11, 91 per cent). Overall, sensitivity was 94 per cent. Several studies have reported sensitivity for maculopathy (Hee *et al.*, 1995) and background retinopathy (Kalm *et al.*, 1989) of around 80 per cent.

Retinal photography Retinal photography is probably the most effective method of screening large widespread populations (Leese *et al.*, 1992). The main advantage is that a permanent record of fundal appearance is obtained. This can be used to document the progression of retinopathy with time, or to observe the effect of treatment. A 35-mm film gives good detail, and stereo photography enables retinal thickening (macular oedema) to be graded. Fundus photography has been shown to improve detection of sight-threatening diabetic retinopathy by optometrists and general practitioners (O'Hare *et al*, 1996; Gibbins *et al*, 1998; Owens *et al*, 1998).

The gold standard of seven-field stereophotography has been accepted as the basis for retinal assessment in many large treatment and intervention trials. However, it is slow and expensive because 14 photographs (seven stereo pairs) need to be taken for each eye, giving 28 photographs in total, and grading takes around 20 minutes for each patient. Many attempts have been made to simplify the procedure. One of these is to take four fields. Moss *et al.* (1989) showed that this only reduced sensitivity by 5 per cent for grading any retinopathy and by 10 per cent for proliferative retinopathy.

With dilated pupils, Harding *et al.* (1995) reported 89 per cent agreement for detecting sight-threatening retinopathy between three fields taken with a non-mydriatic camera and a retinal specialist performing slit lamp BIO.

Kinyoun *et al.* (1989) studied detection of macular oedema. They compared a single 30° stereoscopic fundus photograph centred on the macula, assessed by trained graders, with ophthalmoscopy and slit lamp BIO performed by retinal specialists. The photographs from the Early Treatment Diabetic Retinopathy Study (ETDRS) were used as their template. Macular oedema was graded as yes, no or questionable. Agreement between the retinal specialists and the graders was 78 per cent for oedema within one disc diameter of the centre of the macula, and 83 per cent for hard exudates in the same area. At the first follow-up, agreement was 83 per cent overall. Retinal specialists detected macular oedema in 701 and graders in 650 of 1179 patients. In a later study Kinyoun *et al.* (1992) found 93 per cent agreement between a trained grader and retinal specialist, both grading retinopathy from fundus photographs only.

Retinal photography does have limitations. Cameras are costly, there is a restricted field of view and relatively poor magnification. Polaroid film is widely used but, although the resolution may be sufficient for detecting background diabetic retinopathy, it may be insufficient to detect proliferative diabetic retinopathy. Lack of stereopsis makes detection of macular oedema very difficult. Photographs are easily stored and readable, but the cost of film for each patient is relatively high. Non-mydriatic cameras are not particularly effective in elderly patients with small pupils, and fail to detect lesions outside 45°. With an undilated pupil, image failures can be as high as 27 per cent with non-mydriatic fundus cameras (Ryder *et al.*, 1985). This has led to most screening being carried out with a wide-angle lens through a dilated pupil.

Summary

Several criteria need to be met for a disease to be suitable for screening. All these criteria are met in diabetic retinopathy. Screening programmes are essential if retinopathy is to be effectively treated and morbidity reduced in accord with the St Vincent declaration. The cheapest and most widely available technique is direct ophthalmoscopy; however, it is a relatively insensitive technique. The non-mydriatic camera is a reasonable alternative, and provides a permanent record of the patient's retina. Photography through a dilated pupil gives better results. It is clear that publications over the past 10–15 years addressing the role of photography have raised several different issues for Health Authorities and for specialists in the field of diabetes to consider. The most obvious one is to decide which clinical method, or methods, offers the best rate of detection of sight-threatening retinopathy. Another aspect is that a screening service should not inappropriately refer large numbers of diabetics to the ophthalmology department. Mobile community photographic screening units have been reported as better than ophthalmoscopy in detecting retinopathy (Taylor *et al.*, 1990; Harding *et al.*, 1995, O'Hare *et al.*, 1996). Another promising avenue is to utilize trained optometrists and medical clinical assistants to screen large numbers of patients with slit lamp BIO in order to benefit from the high accuracy that these techniques afford.

The cost-effectiveness of photography and the other modalities must also be considered. Screening in GP health centres has been advocated as a cost-effective method of screening (Rogers *et al.*, 1990; Jacob *et al.*, 1995). The cost per positive case was calculated in a Department of Health Study (Sculpher *et al.*, 1991) and found to vary considerably in the three centres used in the study. The cost per true positive detected by photography was lower with a mobile camera unit taken to general practices than in a hospital-based photography service. Others have addressed costs in terms of the total numbers screened (Harding *et al.*, 1995; O'Hare *et al.*, 1996) and the cost-benefit of additional cases detected if an effective screening programme is introduced.

References

American College of Physicians, American Diabetes Association and American Academy of Ophthalmology (1992). Screening guidelines for diabetic retinopathy (comment). *Ann. Intern. Med.*, **116(8)**, 683–5.

Burns-Cox, C. J. (1996). Prevention of blindness: a lost opportunity (editorial). *J. Medical Screening*, **3(4)**, 169.

Burns-Cox, C. J. and Hart, J. C. (1985). Screening of diabetics for retinopathy by ophthalmic opticians. *Br. Med. J.*, **290**, 1052–4.

Buxton, M. J., Sculpher, M. J., Ferguson, B. A. *et al.* (1991). Screening for treatable diabetic retinopathy: a comparison of different methods. *Diabetic Med.*, **8**, 371–7.

Diabetic Retinopathy Study Research Group (1978). Photocoagulation treatment of proliferative diabetic retinopathy: the second report of diabetic retinopathy study findings. *Ophthalmology*, **85**, 82–105.

Diabetic Retinopathy Study Research Group (1981). Report No. 8. Photocoagulation treatment for proliferative diabetic retinopathy. *Ophthalmology*, **88**, 583–600.

Early Treatment Diabetic Retinopathy Study Group (1985). Report No. 1. Photocoagulation for diabetic macular oedema. *Arch. Ophthalmol.*, **103**, 1796–1806.

Forrest, R. D., Jackson, C. A. and Yudkin, J. S. (1987). Screening for diabetic retinopathy – comparison of a nurse and doctor with retinal photography. *Diabetes* Res., **5**, 39–42.

Gatling, W., Howie, A. J. and Hill, R. D. (1995). An optical practice based diabetic eye screening programme. *Diabetic Med.*, **12(6)**, 531–6.

Gibbins, R. L., Owens, D. R., Allen, J. C. and Eastman, L. (1998). Practical application of the European Field Guide in screening for diabetic retinopathy by using ophthalmoscopy and 35 mm retinal slides. *Diabetologica*, **41(1)**, 59–64.

Hammond, C. J., Shackleton, J., Flanagan, D.W. *et al.* (1996). Comparison between an ophthalmic optician and an ophthalmologist in screening for diabetic retinopathy. *Eye*, **10(1)**, 107–12.

Harding, S. P., Broadbent, D. M., Neoh, C. *et al.* (1995). Sensitivity and specificity of photography and direct ophthalmoscopy in screening for sight-threatening eye disease: the Liverpool Diabetic Eye Study. *Br. Med. J.*, **311(7013)**, 1131–5.

Harris, A., Bonell, C., Evans, T. and Roberson, G. (1994). Commissioning diabetic eye screening by optometrists: a local initiative at the primary–secondary care interface. *J. Medical Screening*, **1(1)**, 13–15.

Hee, M. R., Puliafito, C. A. and Duker, J. S. (1995). Quantitative assessment of macular edema with optical coherence tomography. *Arch. Ophthalmol.*, **113(8)**, 1019–29.

Jacob, J., Stead, J., Sykes, J. *et al.* (1995). A report on the use of technician ophthalmoscopy combined with the use of the Canon non-mydriatic camera in screening for diabetic retinopathy in the community. *Diabetic Med.*, **12**, 419–25.

Javitt, J. C. and Aiello, L. P. (1996). Cost-effectiveness of detecting and treating diabetic retinopathy. *Ann. Intern. Med.*, **124**, 164–9.

Javitt, J. C., Aiello, L. P. and Chiang, T. *et al.* (1994). Preventive eye care in people with diabetes is cost-saving to the federal government. Implications for health-care reform. *Diabetes Care*, **17(8)**, 909–17.

Kalm, H., Egertsen, R. and Blohme, G. (1989). Non-stereo fundus photography as a screening procedure for diabetic retinopathy among patients with Type II diabetes. Compared with 60D enhanced slit-lamp examination. *Acta Ophthalmol.*, **67**, 546–53.

Kinyoun, J. L., Barton, F., Fisher, M. *et al.* (1989). Detection of diabetic macular edema. Ophthalmoscopy versus photography – Early Treatment Diabetic Retinopathy Study Report No. 5. *Ophthalmology*, **96**, 746–51.

Kinyoun, J. L., Martin, D. C., Fujimoto, W. Y. and Leonettie, D. L. (1992). Ophthalmoscopy versus fundus photographs for detecting and grading diabetic retinopathy. *Invest. Ophthalmol. Vis. Sci.*, **33**, 1888–93.

Klein, R. G., Klein, B. E., Moss, S. E. *et al.* (1985a). The Wisconsin Epidemiologic Study of Diabetic Retinopathy. Prevalence and risk of diabetic retinopathy when age at diagnosis is less than 30 years. *Arch Ophthalmol.*, **102**, 520–26.

Klein, R. G., Klein, B. E., Neider, M. W. *et al.* (1985b). Diabetic retinopathy as detected using ophthalmoscopy, a nonmydriatic camera and a standard fundus camera. *Ophthalmology*, **92**, 485–491.

Klein, R. G., Klein, B. E., Moss, S. E. *et al.* (1989). The Wisconsin Epidemiologic Study of Diabetic Retinopathy. IX. Four-year incidence and progression of diabetic retinopathy when age at diagnosis is less than 30 years. *Arch Ophthalmol.*, **107**, 237–43.

Klein, R. G., Klein, B. E. and Moss, S. E. (1990). The Wisconsin Epidemiologic Study of Diabetic Retinopathy: an update. *Aus. NZ J. Ophthalmol.*, **18**, 19–22.

Kohner, E. M. and Porta, M. (1991a). Diabetic retinopathy: preventing blindness in the 1990s (letter). *Diabetologia*, **34(11)**, 844–5.

Kohner, E. M. and Porta, M. (1991b). Protocols for screening and treatment of diabetic retinopathy in Europe. *Eur. J. Ophthalmol.*, **1(1)**, 45–54.

Kristinsson, J. K., Gudmundsson, J. R., Stefansson, E. *et al.* (1995). Screening for diabetic retinopathy. Initiation and frequency. *Acta Ophthalmol. Scand.*, **73(6)**, 525–8.

Leese, G. P., Newton, R. W., Jung, R. T. *et al.* (1992). Screening for diabetic retinopathy in a widely spaced population using non-mydriatic fundus photography in a mobile unit. Tayside Mobile Eye Screening Unit. *Diabetic Med.*, **9(5)**, 459–62.

Leese, G. P., Tesfaye, S., Dengler-Harles, M. *et al.* (1997). Screening for diabetic eye disease by optometrists using slit lamps. *J. R. Coll. Phys.*, **31**, 65–9.

Mitchell, P. and Moffitt, P. (1990). Update and implications from the Newcastle diabetic retinopathy study. *Aus. NZ J. Ophthalmol.*, **18(1),** 13–17.

Moss, S. E., Klein, R. G., Kessler, S. D. and Richie, K. A. (1985). Comparison between ophthalmoscopy and fundus photography in determining severity of diabetic retinopathy. *Ophthalmology,* **93,** 62–7.

Moss, S. E., Meuer, S. M., Klein, R. G. *et al.* (1989). Are seven standard photographic fields necessary for classification of diabetic retinopathy? *Invest. Ophthalmol. Vis. Sci.,* **30,** 823–8.

Newsom, R. (1991). Screening for diabetic retinopathy (letter). *Br. Med. J.,* **302,** 175.

O'Hare, J. P., Hopper, A., Madhaven, C. *et al.* (1996). Adding retinal photography to screening for diabetic retinopathy: a prospective study in the primary care. *Br. Med. J.,* **312,** 679–82.

Owens, D. R., Gibbins, R. L., Lewis, P. A. *et al.* (1998). Screening for diabetic retinopathy by general practitioners: ophthalmoscopy or retinal photography as 35 mm colour transparencies? *Diabetic Med.,* **15(2),** 170–75.

Rogers, D., Bitner-Glindzicz, M., Harris, C. *et al.* (1990). Non-mydriatic retinal photography as a screening service for general practitioners. *Diabetic Med.,* **7,** 165–7.

Ryder, R. E., Young, S., Vora, J. P. *et al.* (1985). Screening for diabetic retinopathy using Polaroid retinal photography through undilated pupils. *Pract. Diabetes,* **2,** 34–9.

Sculpher, M. J., Buxton, M. J., Ferguson, B. A. *et al.* (1991). A relative cost-effectiveness analysis of different methods of screening for diabetic retinopathy. *Diabetic Med.,* **8,** 644–50.

Sussman, E. J., Tsiaras, W. G. and Soper, K. A. (1982). Diagnosis of diabetic eye disease. *JAMA,* **247,** 3231–4.

Taylor, R., Lovelock, L., Tunbridge, W. M. G. *et al.* (1990). Comparison of non-mydriatic retinal photography with ophthalmoscopy in 2159 patients: mobile retinal camera study. *Br. Med. J.,* **301,** 1243–7.

The British Diabetic Association (1994). *Guidelines on the Management of Diabetes in Primary Care.* British Diabetic Association.

Wiek, J., Newsom, R. S. B. and Kohner, E. M. (1991). Role of diabetologists in evaluating diabetic retinopathy (letter). *Diabetes Care,* **14,** 1113.

Williams, R., Nusset, S., Humphrey, R. and Thompson, G. (1986). Assessment of non-mydriatic fundus photography in detection of diabetic retinopathy. *Br. Med. J.,* **293,** 1140–42.

Wilson, J. M. and Junger, Y. G. (1968). Principles of mass screening for disease. *Boletin de la Oficina Sanitaria Panamericana,* **64,** 281–93.

Chapter 10

Applications of fundus photography in diabetic retinopathy

Usha Dhanesha

Introduction

Fundus photography has made a major contribution to understanding the progression of lesions in diabetic retinopathy and to the development of grading systems that offer succinct ways of quantifying the abnormalities seen. Photographic grading schemes have been used to evaluate different methods of screening, predicting the development of advanced stages of the disease and assessing the effects of treatment.

Fundus photography was developed in the nineteenth century. In 1886, Jackman and Webster reported that:

> After considerable practice, and numerous experiments, we have at last succeeded in obtaining a very fair photograph of the blindspot and a few larger blood vessels of the living human retina.

The images were blurred, but this success heralded the production of cameras that could consistently produce high-resolution retinal images. These were based on the Gullstrand principle of reflex-free indirect ophthalmoscopy. However, it took a further half-century to produce a camera that would set the standard for modern instruments. Carbon arc lighting was replaced by electronic flash, and the development of Kodachrome colour film, with exposures of 0.04 s, circumvented problems associated with blinking and eye movements (see Saine, 1996 for detailed review).

Fluorescein and indocyanine angiography

Investigations into the diagnostic use of organic dyes to examine retinal blood flow began following the publication of a method to produce fluorescein sodium (Chopdar, 1989). In 1961, Novotny and Alvis described the intravenous use of fluorescein sodium along with photography to examine the retinal vasculature. The wavelength of peak excitation is about 490 nm, and this is emitted in the yellow-green at about 530 nm. The technique of fluorescein injection and photography has remained virtually unchanged. The patient is positioned in front of the camera and 3–5 ml of 10 per cent sodium is injected into a suitable vein in the lower arm or into the antecubital vein in the space below the elbow. The volume of fluorescein injected depends on the body mass of the patient. Some ophthalmologists prefer to inject a smaller volume of 20 or 25 per cent solution, as this gives better results in eyes with hazy media. It is useful to take a red-free photograph of the retina before the injection in order to obtain a black and white image of the retina and to highlight abnormalities, such as drusen, which may later stain with dye. The dye initially travels to the heart and lungs and appears in the choroidal circulation 3–5 s after the injection. A series of photographs is then taken to document the transit of dye. Five phases are usually distinguished:

1. The pre-arterial phase in which the choroidal circulation fills, resulting in choroidal 'flush'
2. An arterial phase in which the retinal arteries fill with dye
3. A capillary (arteriovenous) phase
4. A venous phase in which the retinal veins fill with dye
5. An after-phase in which dye fades from the retinal and choroidal circulation.

Photographs are taken every few seconds, and the first four phases are completed in about 25 s. After-phase photographs are taken at intervals up to about 20 minutes after the injection to evaluate leaked dye remaining in the retina. Late-phase photographs are therefore important for evaluating diabetic retinopathy. Another injection is needed to obtain photographs of the second eye. Fluorescein dye is excreted slowly, and skin and mucous membranes may stain for a few hours following injection. Urine may be brightly stained for 24–48 hours, and total excretion may take 3 days. Sodium fluorescein is inert, and side-effects are very rare. Approximately 10 per cent of patients may feel nausea for about 30–45 s after the injection, but only a few of these patients actually vomit. Rapid recovery enables late-phase photographs to be taken.

Two principles underlie the diagnostic importance of this technique in assessing diabetic retinopathy. The choroidal blood vessel are fenestrated and fluorescein leaks through vessel walls into the extracellular spaces, causing choroidal flush. The pH of normal blood varies between 7.38 and 7.74, and the intensity of fluorescence is determined by the resulting pH when combined with fluorescein. In the normal retina, the retinal pigment epithelium prevents dye from leaking into the retina from the choroid and dye does not leak out through the retinal vessel walls. In diabetic retinopathy, vascular abnormalities lead either to hyperfluorescence due to dye leaking into the retina or hypofluorescence in areas where perfusion is inadequate. The relative rate at which choroidal and retinal vessels fill with dye in different segments of the fundus may be of clinical importance. Observations during the stages of fluorescein angiography are therefore an invaluable tool in understanding diabetic vascular abnormalities. Stereoscopic fluorescein angiography provides a further means of examining subtle changes in serum accumulation within the retina. It is useful for the ophthalmologist to examine high-resolution colour photographs and fluorescein angiograms side by side in order to identify abnormalities that can be treated with photocoagulation. Recent developments in slit lamp binocular indirect ophthalmoscopy have improved the magnification and definition of fundus examination, and may make fluorescein angiography unnecessary for some patients (Wilkinson, 1986).

Indocyanine green (ICG) can be used to evaluate choroidal vascular abnormalities. This vital dye has a larger molecular weight than fluorescein, and is also administered by injection. ICG binds almost completely to albumin in blood, and does not extravasate out of the choriocapillaries. It therefore delineates blood vessels in the choroid and is particularly useful in identifying subretinal neovascular membranes. A disadvantage is that ICG only emits a small percentage of the incident light in the visible range and a high intensity light source is required for normal photography. This is very uncomfortable for the patient, and exposure time is limited to about 10 s. ICG absorbs and re-emits light in the near infrared at about 805 nm. Observation with an infrared scanning laser ophthalmoscope (SLO) is therefore the method of choice to observe and record staining. Infrared light permits more effective penetration of media opacities and the retinal pigment epithelium. Fluorescein angiography can also be performed with an SLO. A smaller amount of fluorescein is needed for this procedure, and the examination is more comfortable for the patient in terms of light levels. In addition, pupil dilation may not be necessary for all patients.

Photographic methods of recording and grading retinopathy

Different types of photographic film have been used to record retinal images.

Polaroid™ film is useful for obtaining instant hard colour copies. However, Polaroid films are difficult to archive and their relative cost and limited detail have led many researchers to prefer 35 mm transparencies (Williams *et al.*, 1986; Jones *et al.*, 1988; Harding *et al.*, 1995). The poor resolution of Polaroid film may make it difficult to discriminate drusen and exudates. Lesions at the edge of the photograph may have ill-defined margins and appear irregular in shape. Location of macular lesions is aided if the camera has an internal fixation marker. Transparencies offer better resolution than coloured Polaroids, and are traditionally the medium for recording fluorescein angiograms on monochrome film.

Stereo fundus photography

True stereoscopic photography of the fundus entails taking two simultaneous photographs with a slight disparity between them. The images are fused by observing through a stereo slide viewer with positive lenses added to relax accommodation. Grading diabetic retinopathy using stereoscopic pairs was pivotal to research into grading systems such as in the Early Treatment Diabetic Retinopathy Study (ETDRS, 1991). However, true stereo fundus cameras are not in common use, and an alternative proxy method of stereophotography has been developed. This involves taking two images sequentially, with slight disparity between them. An Allen stereo separator is available with Zeiss cameras for this purpose. Most cameras can be used to produce sequential stereo image pairs. This is achieved by moving the camera and illuminating beam slightly to the side for the second photograph. The amount of sideways movement depends on the diameter of the dilated pupil. This method is in wide clinical use.

Pupil dilation is very important in most photographic techniques in order to obtain good image quality and a large field of view. A pupil diameter of more than 4.5 mm is usually recommended.

Fundus cameras are based on the optics of the slit lamp indirect ophthalmoscope, engineered so that an image of the retina is brought to focus on the film (Long, 1991). All fundus cameras have a rheostat for adjusting the illumination, a variable focus, and a range of flash settings. Most cameras offer the following options:

- Polaroid film or 35 mm slide film camera attachments
- variable field of view – as a general guide, the linear magnification varies from approximately 2× for a fundus camera with a 50° field of view to approximately 4× for a 20° field of view.
- auxilliary focusing lenses to compensate for patient's ametropia and/or astigmatism to aid focusing
- external and/or inxternal fixation target
- coloured filters, e.g. green filter for red-free photograph.

The use of fundus photography in the development of grading systems for diabetic retinopathy

Grading is useful for evaluating the progression of diabetic retinopathy, deciding when laser photocoagulation is desirable and in assessing the effects of treatment. One of the first grading systems was used to estimate the effects of pituitary ablation on retinopathy (Joplin *et al.*, 1965). Pituitary ablation was then a recognized treatment for diabetes. The grading system used serial photography to 'reflect changes in component features rather than their absolute severity'. Five components were identified:

- Microaneurysms and haemorrhages
- New vessels
- Venous irregularities

- Hard exudates
- Connective tissue proliferation ('retinitis proliferans').

A four-point grading scale was used: 0, +, ++ or +++.

The grading system was partially qualitative, as it was rare for any feature to be graded +++ at the initial assessment.

In 1967 Oakley *et al.* proposed a more quantifiable grading scale to evaluate the effect of pituitary ablation. This study acknowledged that, although the severity of diabetic retinopathy as a whole passed through stages, individual features advance or regress independently. The same five categories were retained, but five grades of severity were allocated to each feature using four standard photographs. The basis of the gradings was as follows:

- Microaneurysms and haemorrhages – grading according to the number of lesions regardless of size
- New vessels – evaluation of all abnormalities and area of retina involved
- Venous irregularities – percentage of abnormal veins present
- Hard exudates – grading according to the area of retina involved rather than number of lesions
- Connective tissue formation (retinitis proliferans) – grading according to the area involved.

The Airlie House grading system was developed following one of the first meetings to discuss photocoagulation treatment for diabetic retinopathy (Davis *et al.*, 1969). The objective of the Airlie House classification was to provide a simple scheme to express the presence and severity of common fundus lesions. The scheme had to be suitable for both ophthalmoscopic examination and fundus photography. Fourteen lesions were identified and a three-point grading scale used for each:

- Grade 0 – lesion absent
- Grade 1 – mild to moderate
- Grade 2 – severe.

Five standard photographic fields were defined, which included most of the fundus within 30° of the fovea. Predictably, the dividing line between mild to moderate (Grade 1) and severe (Grade 2) was difficult to decide. Written guidelines had to be supplied, and later standard reference photographs were introduced. The panel of experts was aware that the classification would be too complex for some purposes and not detailed enough for others, but suggested that the scheme could be modified to suit individual requirements. In practice it was found to be difficult to achieve agreement between different observers on the presence of the listed abnormalities. This led to the inclusion of a 'questionable category' and then to the development of a five-step grading scale, which subdivided the previous Grade 1 and Grade 2 categories:

- Grade 0 – absent
- Grade 1a – definitely present but less severe than in standard photograph (A)
- Grade 1b – equal to standard photograph (A) but less severe than in standard photograph (B)
- Grade 2a – equal or more severe than in standard photograph (B) but less severe than in standard photograph (C)
- Grade 2b – more severe than in standard photograph (C).

Two additional standard photographic fields were added in the upper and lower nasal quadrants, making seven in all (Figure 10.1; Diabetic Retinopathy Study Research Group, 1981). This scheme of seven fields using stereo fundus photography became the standard procedure for determining the presence and severity of diabetic retinopathy. An optional eighth field was introduced, which was to include the area of retina with the most severe new vessels if not encompassed within fields 1 to 7.

The seven-field standard system was further modified by Klein *et al.* (1984) to include six grades or levels to help identify progression of retinopathy after 2 years and at a 6-year follow-up. Standard photographs were provided as a

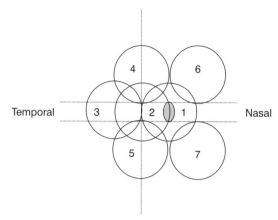

Figure 10.1 Schematic representation of the seven fields utilised by the DRS (1981). Shaded oval represents the optic disc.

guide. This grading scheme aimed to characterize overall progression, and was most useful in clinical trials designed to assess treatment. In fact, the researchers found a greater prevalence of retinopathy (60 per cent) after 5–10 years duration of diabetes than other studies, and attributed this to the sensitivity of the grading system. However, grading individual features was very labour intensive. Seven stereo pairs had to be obtained for each eye, and evaluation was time consuming. The reproducibility of grading by different observers also had to be addressed. This was dealt with by having the baseline photographs of each patient independently assessed by four individuals and the differences resolved by discussion. A second measure of reproducibility was estimated by randomly selecting photos from the 2- and 6-year follow-up data and grading these photos independently without the grader having access to photographs from the fellow eye or other visits. Two additional methods were devised to assess the overall severity of retinopathy by referring to the level in the worst eye and the retinopathy level in each eye. The latter was found to increase the sensitivity by which progression was identified. It was found that level 4 grading, which included haemorrhages, cotton wool spots, IRMA and/or venous beading, was of prognostic importance for the relatively small number of diabetic patients in

this study. A patient with level 4 retinopathy in each eye at baseline progressed to proliferative retinopathy in at least one eye at the 6-year examination. If two lesions were assigned level 4 gradings, then the risk of progression to proliferative diabetic retinopathy was 23 per cent.

Grading maculopathy

The grading of maculopathy was also initiated so that the effects of photocoagulation at the posterior pole could be assessed (ETDRS, 1985). Both fluorescein angiography and baseline fundus photography were used to identify the patient group, and clinically significant macula oedema was defined as:

- retinal thickening within 500 μm of the fovea
- hard exudates within 500 μm of the fovea
- an area of retinal thickening larger than one disc area, any part of which is within one disc diameter of the fovea.

A distance of 500 μm is approximately equivalent to one-third of the disc diameter (see Chapters 5 and 6).

Another grading scheme was devised by Aldington et al. (1995), based on the 45° field obtained with a non-mydriatic camera. This involved two photographic fields; a macular field positioned so that the exact centre of the optic disc lay at the nasal end of the horizontal meridian of the field of view, and a second field where the optic disc was positioned one disc diameter from the temporal edge of the field along the horizontal meridian. The grading of the different lesions contained in each field contributed to the calculation of an overall retinopathy level. The concept behind this was that groups of lesions that occur together are broad indicators of progression towards proliferative retinopathy. This scheme was thought to be useful for large epidemiological studies, but could not be fully assessed or compared with other grading methods because stereo photography was not used and only a limited area of the retina was visualized.

Summary

Grading systems based on photography can be modified to suit different project designs and provide a basis for multicentre research. Complex grading systems based on stereoscopic photographs were mainly used to assess the efficacy of treatments such as pituitary ablation and, later, panretinal and focal laser photocoagulation (Klein *et al.*, 1990). The success of photocoagulation is now well established. The same grading systems contributed to epidemiological studies, and established that the onset and progression of retinopathy was associated with increasing duration of diabetes. Serial photography over a number of years identified the combination of lesions that predicts the rate of progression to proliferative retinopathy and maculopathy (ETDRS, 1991). The ETDRS standard photographs were used by ophthalmologists and trained photographic graders to identify the stage at which laser treatment is most beneficial. Grading systems which are most useful for optometric shared care schemes need not be so detailed. It is important to be able to estimate the possible speed of progression and hence to vary the intervals between follow-up examinations. Secondly, criteria for referral to an ophthalmologist need to be identified – not only when treatment is needed, but when rapid progression is anticipated or when assessment with other more detailed techniques such as fluorescein angiography is required.

Different health authorities and health commissioning groups will address the issue of screening for sight-threatening retinopathy in a number of different ways. Photography has a role in the context of screening in the provision of photographs that can serve as visual documentation, in trying to quantify the level of the condition and in contributing information to a database.

Within this context grading of retinopathy can provide an effective communication tool, and the provision of a photograph provides a permanent objective record of written documentation. Photography can also be of value in clinical audit of screening programmes, analysis of detection rates, appropriateness of referral and in monitoring treatments.

Historically grading of retinopathy has evolved through the medium of fundus photography, and this cannot be underestimated in its value as an important technique by which retinopathy can be assessed in a quantitative way that complements the use of ophthalmoscopy and biomicroscopic fundus examination.

References

Aldington, S. J., Kohner, E. M., Meuer, S. *et al.* (1995). Methodology for retinal photography and assessment of diabetic retinopathy: the EURODIAB IDDM complications study. *Diabetologia*, **38**, 437–44.

Chopdar, A. (1989). *Manual of Fundus Photography.* Butterworth-Heinemann.

Davis, M. D., Norton, E. W. D. and Myers, F. L. (1969). The Airlie classification of diabetic retinopathy. In: *Symposium on the Treatment of Diabetic Retinopathy* (M. F. Goldberg and S. L. Fine, eds), pp. 7–22. US Government Printing Office, USPHS Publ. No. 1890.

Diabetic Retinopathy Study Research Group (1981). Report No. 7. A modification of the Airlie House classification of diabetic retinopath. *Invest. Ophthalmol. Vis. Sci.*, **21**, 210–26.

Early Treatment Diabetic Retinopathy Study Report (1985). Report No. 1. Photocoagulation for diabetic macular oedema. *Arch. Ophthalmol.*, **103**, 1796–1806.

Early Treatment Diabetic Retinopathy Study Research Group (1991). Report No. 12. Fundus photographic risk factors for progression of diabetic retinopathy. *Ophthalmology*, **98**, 823–33.

Harding, S. P., Broadbent, D. M., Neoh, C. *et al.* (1995). Sensitivity and specificity of photography and direct ophthalmoscopy in screening for sight-threatening eye disease: the Liverpool diabetic study. *Br. Med. J.*, **311**, 1131–5.

Jackman, W. T. and Webster, J. D. (1886). On photographing the retina of the living eye. *Philadelphia Chronicle*, **23**, 275.

Jones, D., Dolben, J., Owens, D. R. *et al.* (1988). Non-mydriatic Polaroid photography in screening for diabetic retinopathy: Evaluation in a clinical setting. *Br. Med. J.*, **296**, 1029–30.

Joplin, G. F., Fraser, R., Hill, D. W. *et al.* (1965) Pituitary ablation for diabetic retinopathy. *Q. J. Med.*, **XXXIV**, 443–62.

Klein, B. E. K., Davis, M. D., Segal, P. *et al.* (1984). Diabetic retinopathy: assessment of severity and progression. *Ophthalmology*, **91**, 10–17.

Klein, R., Klein, B. E. K. and Moss, S. E. (1990). The Wisconsin Epidemiologic Study of Diabetic Retinopathy; an update. *Aus. NZ J. Ophthalmol.*, **18**, 19–22.

Long, W. F. (1991). Fundus photography. In: *Clinical Procedures in Optometry* (J. B. Eskridge, J. F. Amos and J. D. Bartlett, eds), pp. 334–44. JB Lippincott Co.

Novotny, H. R. and Alvis, D. L. (1961). A method of photographing fluorescent circulating blood in the human retina. *Circulation*, **24**, 82–6.

Oakley, N., Hill, D. W., Jopling, F. *et al.* (1967). The assessment of severity and progression by comparison with a set of standard fundus photographs. *Diabetologia*, **3**, 402–5.

Saine, P. J. (1996). Landmarks in the development of fundus photography. In: *Ophthalmic Photography* (P. J. Siane and M. E. Tyler, eds). Butterworth-Heinemann.

Wilkinson, C. P. (1986). Limitation and over-utilisation of angiographic services. *Ophthalmology*, **93**, 401–4.

Williams, R., Nusset, S., Humphrey, R. and Thompson, G. (1986). Assessment of non-mydriatic fundus photography in detection of diabetic retinopathy. *Br. Med. J.*, **293**, 1140–42.

Chapter 11

Digital imaging of diabetic retinopathy
Christopher G. Owen

Introduction

Methods of identification of diabetic retino-pathy usually involve visual recognition of specific retinal features using binocular indi-rect ophthalmoscopy (BIO). Alternatively, visual recognition can be performed from pho-tographic prints, transparencies or digital images. These methods rely upon an agreed method of classification, which was men-tioned in Chapter 10. Developments in digital imaging allow computerized assessment of fundus images using algorithms designed to detect certain retinal structures such as blood vessels or aneurysms. More recently, neural networks have been employed to enable the computer to learn to identify distinctive fea-tures of diabetic retinopathy from a series of images.

Polaroid™ film has the advantage of almost instant development, but the image quality is inferior to 35 mm colour transparencies. The main disadvantage of colour transparencies is the delay between photographing the fundus and viewing the images. Usually many patients' fundi are recorded on one film, which then has to be developed before the images can be viewed individually. Digital cameras offer instantaneous images that can be viewed directly on a computer monitor and can be magnified, digitally enhanced and stored on a computer. Digital images are comparable in quality visually to colour transparencies. If necessary, stored images can be sent elsewhere via e-mail for evaluation visually or by com-puter. Printed copies can be made using high-resolution colour printers.

The emergence of digital imaging in med-ically related fields has been rapid and multi-functional. This chapter introduces the ter-minology associated with digital imaging and describes the application of the technique to the detection of diabetic retinopathy. A number of digital fundus cameras are described, and their future applications are discussed.

What is a digital image?

A digital image can be thought of as a two-dimensional light intensity function $f(x,y)$, where x,y denotes a spatial co-ordinate in the image and f corresponds to the brightness or colour content at that point. The digital image can be considered as a matrix of picture elements m wide and n deep. The term picture elements is often abbreviated to '*pixels*'.

$$f(x,y) = \begin{bmatrix} f(0,0) & f(0,1) & f(0,m-1) \\ f(1,0) & f(1,1) & f(1,m-1) \\ \vdots & & \vdots \\ f(n-1,0)f(n-1,1)\cdots f(n-1,m-1) \end{bmatrix}$$

Treating an image in this way allows areas of interest to be extracted or enhanced using mathematical techniques to transform the image function. This numerical format is advantageous in that it permits images to be stored or transmitted electronically.

Digital images are formed by physical de-vices that are sensitive to a narrow band of the

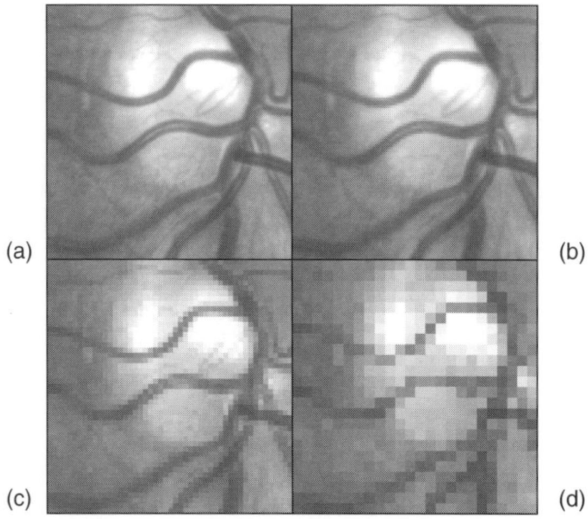

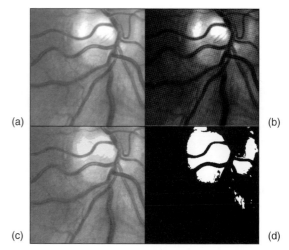

Figure 11.1 Sampling levels (a) 200×200 pixels; (b) 100×100; (c) 50×50 and (d) 25×25.

Figure 11.2 Brightness levels (a) 24-bit image with 16.7 million grey levels; (b) 8-bit with 256 grey levels; (c) 4-bit with 16 grey levels; and (d) 1-bit with two grey levels.

electromagnetic energy spectrum and produce an electrical signal proportional to the level of energy detected. Digital cameras contain a number of photosites, each of which produces a voltage proportional to the intensity of the incident light. A series of photosites is known collectively as a charged couple device (CCD). The number of photosites contained within a CCD of a digital camera is described as the pixel resolution. Image quality declines as the pixel resolution is reduced (Figure 11.1).

A monochrome digital imaging device produces a signal divided into k equal brightness steps. This brightness value is expressed in bits (b) where $k = 2^b$. An 8-bit image contains 256 brightness levels, a 4-bit image 16 levels, and a 1-bit (binary) image two brightness levels. Figure 11.2 shows the effect of reducing the number of brightness levels in an image. Visually there is very little difference between images with 16.7 million levels of brightness (24-bit image) and 256 levels of brightness; however, an image with 16 brightness levels begins to show degradation.

A monochrome image is unlikely to have sufficient information to identify the features of diabetic retinopathy, and colour images are needed. Colour reproduction is achieved in

digital cameras by using three sensors sensitive to a narrow band of wavelengths in the red, green and blue parts of the visual spectrum. Signals from each sensor are processed and combined to achieve a full colour image. Colour images require more storage capacity than monochromatic images, but this does not usually present a problem with modern computer hardware.

Some fundus features are not best observed using light of a broad spectrum of wavelengths. Delori *et al.* (1977) found using illumination between 540 and 580 nm was best for looking at the retinal vasculature. Optimal visualization of vasculature was observed with a narrow band of wavelengths at about 570 nm (yellow-green). Ducrey *et al.* (1979) stated that:

> restriction of the spectral content of illumination to an appropriate narrow spectral band or the use of monochromatic light improves both contrast and optical quality over that obtained with white light and results in enhanced visualization of [vascular] structures.

Hence many fundus cameras utilize green (red-free) imaging to optimize contrast between vessels and the surrounding retina. This can be achieved by using the signal from the green sensor of the CCD array alone, taking images with a red-free filter (green filter), or both.

Digital cameras can also be used to digitize colour transparencies and photographs. Remky et al. (1996) found that using the green sensor alone to digitize colour fundus photographs provided images with superior contrast for measuring the width of blood vessels in diabetic fundi before and after panretinal laser photocoagulation.

Most of the currently available digital fundus cameras have red-free imaging options (Table 11.1). It is noteworthy that human colour vision and digital camera colour sensitivity do not correspond exactly, and a filter which gives the best visual contrast may not be the best to use in a digital system.

Digital camera systems for fundus imaging

There are a number of fundus cameras that provide digital imaging. Examples are listed in Table 11.1. Some require mydriasis while others do not, provided the pupil is of sufficient size. Hand-held devices are also available, which are ideally suited to outreach clinics (Nidek Handy NM100, Birmingham Optical Group; Kowa Genesis, Keeler).

Each camera system consists of an optical configuration that splits the fundus image into two channels, a viewing system and an image sensor. The image sensor can be photographic, video analogue or digital. Digital camera systems with higher pixel resolutions are associated with images of superior quality. This is a great advantage in identifying and distinguishing features of diabetic retinopathy, especially when the image is enlarged and viewed on a high-resolution monitor. There are various software options for viewing digital images. Some are dedicated to a camera system, such as IMAGEnet used with Topcon cameras, others such as OCUlab PRO (Life Science Resource) are interchangeable. Most software offers image enhancement, image optimization and compar-

ative quantitative measurement. Measurements include CD ratios or the size of a feature in pixels or compared with the size of the individual's disc. Comparative measurements in the same eye are always useful, but practitioners should beware of systems that claim to measure 'true size'. This can only be achieved if the patient's refractive error is known and measurements of corneal curvature and axial length are made to determine the magnification of the eye (Bennett et al., 1994).

Digital imaging methods for monitoring diabetic retinopathy

Recent studies show that digital images are superior to Polaroid film in quality, but are not as yet superior in visual quality to 35 mm colour transparencies.

Ryder et al. (1998) compared the diagnostic capability of digital and Polaroid images, taken with a Cannon CR5 45NM, for 58 eyes with diabetic retinopathy. Diabetic retinopathy was correctly diagnosed from digital images in 95 per cent of cases (n = 55/58) and from Polaroid film in 84 per cent of cases (n = 49/58). All 34 eyes with diabetic retinopathy requiring referral to an ophthalmologist were correctly identified from digital images, but only 24 eyes (71 per cent) were identified from Polaroid film. Side by side comparisons revealed much better resolution of retinal features in the digital image format. Using the same type of camera, George et al. (1998) compared two-field 45° digital images with colour transparencies. The diagnosis of diabetic retinopathy agreed in 70 of the 75 eyes examined (93 per cent). Overall, one eye was overgraded and four eyes were undergraded. In two of those undergraded IRMA were not identified, possibly due to inadequate image resolution, and in another eye small cotton wool spots were incorrectly diagnosed as laser photocoagulation scars in the digital image.

George et al. (1997) digitized 150 retinal 35 mm colour transparencies to a resolution of 768×512 pixels and displayed the images on a monitor with a resolution of 800×600 pixels.

Table 11.1 Some of the fundus digital imaging systems currently available

Model	Field of view	Imaging media	Image options	Pupil	Digital camera (pixel resolution)	Image software
Topcon TRC-50EX	20°, 35°, 50°	Polaroid/film/video/digital	Red-free, fluorescein angiography, colour	> 4.5 mm	Kodak Megaplus (1024×1024)/Sony DCX950P (800×600)	IMAGEnet software, allows storage, viewing and analysis
Topcon TRC-50IX	20°, 35°, 50°	Polaroid/film/video/digital	Red-free, fluorescein angiography, ICG, colour	> 4.5 mm	Kodak Megaplus (1024×1024)/Sony DCX950P (800×600)	IMAGEnet software
Topcon TRC-NW5S Still video	20°, 45°	Digital/video	Colour	> 4.0 mm	Sony DCX950P (800×600)	IMAGEnet software
Cannon CF-60 UVi	30°, 40°, 60°	Polaroid/film/digital	Red-free, fluorescein angiography, ICG, colour	> 4.0 mm	Hitachi HV-C20 (800×600)	Retinal Imaging Systems 98 software
Cannon CR6-45NM	30°, 45°	Polaroid/film/digital	Red-free, colour	> 3.7 mm	Sony DCX950P (800×600)	Retinal Imaging Systems Lite 98 software
Cannon CF-60 UD	40°, 60°	Polaroid/film/digital	Red-free, colour	> 4.0 mm	Hitachi HV-C20 (800×600)	Retinal Imaging Systems 98 software

Retinopathies were graded independently from both transparencies and monitor. Compared to recognition from colour transparencies, 84 of 88 eyes with sight-threatening diabetic retinopathy (95 per cent) and 62 eyes with non-sight-threatening diabetic retinopathy (100%) were correctly diagnosed from the monitor. The most likely reason for the disagreement is the reduced resolution of the monitor compared with photographic film.

Sony and Hitachi digital cameras used with the Canon and Topcon fundus cameras have similar pixel resolutions. The rapid development of digital cameras has produced equipment that can provide resolutions of 1024 ×1024 pixels (Kodak Megaplus). However, an increase in pixel resolution is of little consequence if the image is displayed on a monitor or imaging package with a lower resolution. Currently monitors are available which have resolutions of 1600×1000 pixels. It is therefore only a matter of time before digital fundus images will have superior resolution to colour transparencies.

Application and future uses of digital imaging

A digital image can be considered as numerical information that can be manipulated mathematically. Image processing can enhance contrast and remove noise within an image. Image segmentation is a different procedure from enhancement, and is the process of performing foreground/background separation. Segmentation is the first step in extracting regions of interest, such as individual blood vessel or hard exudates, and enables specific structures to be identified, quantified and monitored for progression. Edge detection plays an important role in a number of image-processing applications, and is used to locate boundaries or sharp gradients within the image function. Several studies have used edge detection techniques to segment retinal blood vessels from the surrounding retina (Tamura *et al.*, 1988; Chaudhuri *et al.*, 1989; Zhou *et al.*, 1994). Similar imaging techniques have been applied to other

vascular beds, such as those in the conjunctiva (Villumsen *et al.*, 1991), heart (Shmueli *et al.*, 1983; Pappas and Lim, 1988) and cochlea (Miles and Nuttall, 1993). There are other non-medical applications.

In recent years artificial neural networks have emerged as a useful tool, with a number of clinical applications. Input of prediagnosed normal and abnormal data 'teaches' the computer to recognize and extract specific abnormalities from new images. The sensitivity and specificity of the network depends on the quality, variety and volume of data input and on the quality of new images to be analysed. A neural network has already been used to identify Type 2 diabetes in obese patients (Bardini *et al.*, 1998; Su, 1994).

Gardner *et al.* (1996) employed a neural network to identify retinopathy in diabetic patients. Red-free fundus photographs of the posterior pole were obtained for 200 diabetic patients and 101 normals. The images were digitized to a 700×700 pixel square and then subdivided into 30×30 and 20×20 pixel elements. Detection rates for the recognition of blood vessels, exudates, and haemorrhages were 92 per cent, 93 per cent and 74 per cent respectively. Overall, the neural network achieved a sensitivity of 88 per cent and specificity of 84 per cent compared with the diagnosis of an ophthalmologist.

Summary

The infrastructure for identifying diabetic patients with retinopathy who would benefit from treatment is not universally available (Williamson and Keating, 1998). Either more resources are needed or existing resources need to be used more effectively. Digital images are instant and readily stored, and can be enhanced and electronically transmitted via e-mail. Diagnosis could be made at remote hospital centres, either by a specially trained observer or by a dedicated diagnostic neural network. It has been estimated that the widespread use of neural networks to diagnose diabetic retinopathy from digital images could reduce the number of patients requiring specialist examination by 70 per cent (Gardner *et al.*, 1996). The lack of personal observation is still viewed by many as an alien concept, but taking part in a computerized diagnostic scheme with electronic links may well be attractive to some co-management teams. The use of telemedicine in the diagnosis of diabetic retinopathy and glaucoma has already emerged (Marcus *et al.*, 1998), although its practice was associated with some expertise. In this study an ophthalmoscope was fitted with a digital micro-camera and the images were transmitted in real time to a reviewing ophthalmologist. The next decade is likely to see an evolution in the monitoring of diabetic retinopathy using digital imaging systems.

References

Bardini, G., Mannucci, E., Ognibene, A. *et al.* (1998). The use of neural networks in the screening for diabetes in obese patients. *Diabetologia*, **41(S1)**, 458.

Bennett, A. G., Rudnicka, A. R. and Edgar, D. F. (1994). Improvements on Littmann's method of determining the size of retinal features by fundus photography. *Grafes Arch. Clin. Exp. Ophthalmol.*, **232**, 361–7.

Chaudhuri, S., Chatterjee, S., Katz, N. *et al.* (1989). Detection of blood vessels in retinal images using two-dimensional matched filters. *IEEE Trans. Med. Imag.*, **8(3)**, 263–9.

Delori, F. C., Gragoudas, E. S., Francisco, R. and Pruett, R. C. (1977). Monochromatic ophthalmoscopy and fundus photography: the normal fundus. *Arch. Ophthalmol.*, **95**, 861–8.

Ducrey, N. M., Delori, F. C. and Gragoudas, E. S. (1979). Monochromatic ophthalmoscopy and fundus photography: the pathological fundus. *Arch. Ophthalmol.*, **97**, 288–93.

Gardner, G. G., Keating, D., Williamson, T. H. and Elliott, A. T. (1996). Automatic detection of diabetic retinopathy using a artificial neural network: a screening tool. *Br. J. Ophthalmol.*, **80**, 940–44.

George, L. D., Leverton, C., Young, S. *et al.* (1997). Can digitised colour 35 mm transparencies be used to diagnose diabetic retinopathy? *Diabetic* Med., **14(11)**, 970–73.

George, L. D., Halliwell, M., Hill, R. *et al.* (1998). A comparison of digital retinal images and 35 mm colour transparencies in detecting and grading diabetic retinopathy. *Diabetic Med.*, **15(3)**, 250–53.

Marcus, D. M., Brooks, S. E., Ulrich, L. D. *et al.* (1998). Telemedicine diagnosis of eye disorders by direct ophthalmoscopy – a pilot study. *Ophthalmology*, **105(10)**, 1907–14.

Miles, F. P. and Nuttall, A. L. (1993). Matched filter estimation of serial blood vessel diameters from video images. *IEEE Trans. Med. Imag.*, **12(2)**, 147–52.

Pappas, T. N. and Lim, J. S. (1988). A new method for estimation of coronary artery dimensions in angiograms. *IEEE Trans. Acoustics Speech Signal Processing*, **36(9)**, 1501–13.

Remky, A., Arend, O., Beassencourt, E. *et al.* (1996). Vessel diameter changes before and after panretinal laser photocoagulation in diabetic retinopathy. A method using digitized colour fundus slides. *Klin. Monats. Augenheilkunde*, **209(2–3)**, 79–83.

Ryder, R. E. J., Kong, N., Bates, A. S. *et al.* (1998). Instant electronic imaging systems are superior to Polaroid at detecting sight-threatening diabetic retinopathy. *Diabetic Med.*, **15(3)**, 254–8.

Shmueli, K., Brody, W. R. and Macovski, A. (1983). Estimation of blood vessel boundaries in X-ray images. *Opt. Eng.*, **22(1)**, 110–16.

Su, M. C. (1994). Use of neural networks as medical diagnosis expert systems. *Computers Biol. Med.*, **24(6)**, 419–29.

Tamura, S., Okamato, Y. and Yanashima, K. (1988). Zero-crossing interval correction in tracing eye-fundus blood vessels. *Pattern Recog.*, **21(3)**, 227–33.

Villumsen, J., Ringquist, J. and Alm, A. (1991). Image analysis of conjunctival hyperaemia: a personal computer based system. *Acta. Ophthalmol.*, **69**, 536–9.

Williamson, T. H. and Keating, D. (1998). Telemedicine and computers in diabetic retinopathy screening. *Br. J. Ophthalmol.*, **82**, 5–7.

Zhou, L., Rzeszotarski, M. S., Singerman, L. J. and Chokeff, J. M. (1994). The detection and quantification of retinopathy using digital angiograms. *IEEE Trans. Med. Imag.*, **13(4)**, 619–26.

Chapter 12

Slit lamp biomicroscopic fundus examination

Alicja Rudnicka

Introduction

Slit lamp binocular indirect ophthalmoscopy (BIO) or indirect fundus biomicroscopy has revolutionized the examination of the internal ocular structures. It allows a stereoscopic view of the vitreous cavity and retina, and is considered the standard clinical technique for examining diabetic fundi. Condensing lenses are hand-held and can be either contact or non-contact. The contact variety produce an erect magnified fundus image, and non-contact lenses produce a real, inverted and laterally reversed image. Both techniques benefit from stereopsis and, unlike direct ophthalmoscopy, a good view can be obtained in patients with high degrees of ametropia and the image is less affected by media opacities. With the indirect viewing system the natural pupil is eliminated as a field stop; thus a wide field of view is possible. There are many commercially available condensing lenses, but this chapter will deal with those mainly used in the clinical setting. Table 12.1 summarizes the properties of some condensing lenses available from Volk (Volk Optical Inc. USA). The majority of the lenses are made from high index glass and are double aspheric in construction. As with other indirect lenses, the lower powered condensing lenses produce greater magnification. The higher the power of the lens, the smaller the magnification and working distance, but the larger the field of view. Magnification can be further adjusted by changing the slit lamp biomicroscope magnification setting, and the

magnification and field of view are also governed by the design and diameter of the condensing lens. Table 12.1 gives static and dynamic fields of view. The former is the field of view achieved with the Volk lens held stationary, and the latter is the increased field of view obtained if the Volk lens is moved to bring other areas of the fundus into view. The values quoted in Table 12.1 are approximate and calculated for an emmetropic eye. The real values depend upon the working distance, lens design, patient's ametropia and the skill of the practitioner.

The +60D, +78D and +90D lenses were the first generation to be manufactured by Volk and have a symmetrical double aspheric optical design. They can be held with either surface facing the patient. The 60D provides the highest magnification, and is useful for examining the macula and optic disc. The +78D lens is a good general lens, having a field of view comparable to the +90D but with a higher magnification. The Super66™ is designed for high magnification viewing of the macula region. Although its magnification is similar to the +60D, it offers a superior field of view, and the manufacturing literature states that the Super66 lens gives better resolution, image clarity and depth perception.

The SuperField™ has the same magnification as the +90D, but the lens diameter is larger and hence it offers a wider field of view. Some practitioners prefer the larger size as it is easier to manipulate the lens in the orbital area of the eye. The SuperPupil™ has the widest field of

Table 12.1 Characteristics of a selection of Volk lenses for non-contact indirect fundus biomicroscopy

Lens type	Lens diameter (mm)	Approximate field of view (static/dynamic)	Approximate working distance from cornea (mm)	Approximate linear magnification
+60D	31	67°/81°	12	1.15
Super 66	31	80°/88°	11	1.00
+78D	31	73°/87°	7	0.87
+90D	21.5	74°/89°	7	0.76
SuperField	27	95°/116°	7	0.76
SuperPupil	16	103°/124°	2 to 4	0.45

view, and was designed to be used with undilated/miotic pupils. Of the lenses in Table 12.1, it certainly offers the best field of view through an undilated pupil, and was marketed as the lens of choice in patients in whom it is inadvisable to dilate the pupil.

Some of the indirect lenses have additional attachments:

- a lid adapter to assist with holding of the lid
- a multi-AR coated yellow filter designed to protect the retina during prolonged fundus examinations and provide better patient comfort; however, this can lead to misinterpretation of optic disc pallor and macula oedema
- a contact adapter which converts the optical set-up in to a direct viewing system
- a retinal scale to allow comparative measurements to be made of retinal features – this can only be used to reliably monitor changes within one patient but not to compare measurements across patients, and the scale of measurement will vary with ametropia, working distance and lens design.

This list is not exhaustive; other attachments exist to change the magnification and field of view.

As slit lamp BIO is the method of choice for routine examination of the diabetic fundus, this will be described in some detail below. Direct contact fundus biomicroscopy is not described here as it is not advisable for routine examination of diabetic patients because of the risk of inducing corneal epithelial abrasions.

Examination procedure

The technique of indirect fundus biomicroscopy is similar for all lenses. The guidelines given below are designed to help novices master this method; however, there is no substitute for practical experience. In general, it is preferable to perform slit lamp BIO in a darkened room. It is imperative that the usual slit lamp adjustments are made for the examiner's refraction, pupillary distance, and the chin rest height for the patient. Condensing lenses should be kept as clean as possible to minimize disturbing reflections and aberrations.

Initial setting-up

1. The patient's pupils should be maximally dilated, as this increases the field of view and improves image clarity. It is noteworthy that, with experience, a reasonably proficient examination can be performed without dilation in patients with naturally large pupils which do not miose aggressively during fundus biomicroscopy.
2. Illumination and observation systems of the slit lamp biomicroscope should be aligned (zero displacement).
3. The slit beam should be of medium width, of low to medium light intensity and

mid-height. Set the slit lamp biomicroscope magnification to no more than 16×. With higher magnifications it is more difficult to keep a check on the orientation and position relative to the patient.

4. Direct the patient to view a target straight ahead with the eye not under examination.

There are two ways of starting the slit lamp BIO, and each method will now be described in turn.

Methods of viewing

Method A Focus the slit lamp light beam on the patient's pupil. Looking from the side of the instrument, place the condensing lens in front of the patient's eye by holding it between the thumb and forefinger. It should be carefully centred in front of the cornea, with the back surface 6–10 mm from the corneal apex, so that a section of light can be seen in the cornea and entering the crystalline lens. The hand holding the lens can be rested against the forehead strap or side portion of the slit lamp head support and/or on the patient's cheek and brow. Keeping the lens stable, move to look through the slit lamp eyepieces. At this point the view through the eyepieces will appear dark and featureless. Pull the slit lamp slowly away from the patient, maintaining a straight path. Gradually a red glow from the fundus appears and, as the slit lamp is pulled back further, the red blur will focus and the retina will come into view. This is difficult to perform initially as it requires the lens to be held in a stable position and the slit lamp to be pulled straight back without any lateral movement. The total excursion is about 2.5 cm.

Method B Place the slit lamp as far back as possible from the patient and ensure the room lights are dimmed as this will help to locate the path of light from the slit lamp. With the patient looking straight ahead, centre the condensing lens in front of the cornea at a vertex distance of approximately 6–10 mm. Alter the lateral position of the slit lamp so that it is aligned with the lens. Looking from the side of

the instrument, if the slit lamp is indeed aligned with the condensing lens, the examiner should be able to visualize the light entering the patient's pupil. This can be made easier by widening and increasing the illumination of the slit lamp light beam. However, before proceeding it must be returned to the settings described in step 3 above to avoid discomfort to the patient. Keeping the lens in a stable position, move to look through the slit lamp eyepieces. At this point the view through the eyepieces will appear dark and featureless. Push the slit lamp forward slowly towards the patient, maintaining a straight path. Gradually a red glow from the fundus will come into view and, as the slit lamp is moved nearer to the patient, the red blur will focus and the retina will appear.

Improving the view Once a view of the fundus has been achieved it is useful to check the lateral and vertical position of the lens to see if the image quality can be improved. In particular, the vertex distance of the lens from the eye effects both the field of view and image clarity.

If there are disturbing reflections it maybe that the condensing lens is not perpendicular to the patient's eye. Tilting the lens can help; alternatively, the illumination system of some slit lamps can be tilted forward to avoid disturbing reflections. Condensing lens should be kept as clean as possible.

Check binocularity by closing each eye in turn and compare the view. If the view is not binocular or is asymmetrical, check the lateral position of the condensing lens and move it in the direction of the eye not seeing the full picture. Stereopsis is not always achieved immediately, but ensuring the slit lamp biomicroscope is correctly set up at the start is important. For difficulties with fusion, check the position of the eyepieces and ametropia setting on the slit lamp. Occasionally altering the tilt of one's head can help with fusion. The optic disc is a good starting point to practice viewing stereoscopically, as depth should be appreciated when observing the optic cup and retinal vessels as they leave and enter the optic disc.

Hold the condensing lens with left hand to examine a patient's right eye and *vice versa*. A lens mount is available that attaches to the side of the head support of the slit lamp, therefore freeing the hands for other tasks, such as more complex slit lamp examination techniques or laser treatment. Alternatively, a lens mounted extension ring that rests against the patient's brow can be used to steady the lens.

Examining other parts of the fundus

Slit lamp BIO is a dynamic procedure, and lateral and/or vertical adjustments to both the lens and slit lamp position are needed to examine other areas of the fundus. The amount of movement required is relatively small, but the speed of movement of light across the fundus will appear quite fast and in the opposite direction. With most indirect lenses, a wide region of the fundus can be examined with the patient's gaze in the primary position and by moving the light beam and lens to maximize the field of view. The magnification and beam width may also be adjusted as desired. If the beam is too narrow only a thin section of light illuminates the retina, which is not particularly useful. Widening the beam width will increase the area of retina illuminated and thus the area viewed is enlarged, but if the beam is too wide this can degrade image quality as reflections are emphasized. Increasing the beam width/illumination may be

uncomfortable for the patient. It requires practice to complete a full fundus examination successfully. It is best to adopt a systemic approach that ensures all areas of posterior pole are examined.

As with direct ophthalmoscopy, more anterior retinal structures can be examined by altering the patient's direction of gaze and re-positioning the condensing lens. Alignment is important for maintaining a clear stereoscopic view.

The patient should be encouraged to blink normally but to hold the eyes as wide open as possible between blinks. If a patient is unable to hold the eye open wide enough, it may be useful to retract the upper lid with the fourth finger. If a patient has unsteady fixation, it is difficult to keep the image of the fundus in focus. Providing a clearly visible fixation target for the eye that is not under examination can help maintain steady fixation. If a patient is particularly photophobic, reduce the light intensity, beam width and height.

Interpretation of fundal view and recording

It is not easy to adapt to the inverted and laterally reversed image as shown in Figure 12.1a and b; however, locating the optic disc will help with orientation. If the patient is looking up, the superior quadrant of the retina is illuminated but the image of the superior

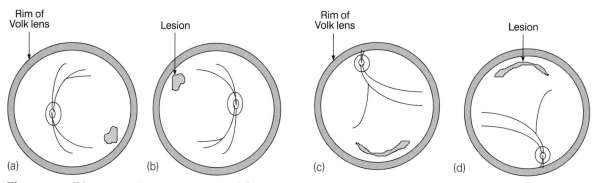

Figure 12.1 Diagrammatic representation of the view and interpretation of ocular fundus with indirect biomicroscopy. (a) View of posterior pole of right eye through indirect lens; (b) true location of features; (c) view of superior fundus through indirect lens with patient looking upwards; (d) true location of features.

fundus is upside down and laterally reversed. Thus, the disc is seen at the upper edge of the field of view of the superior quadrant (Figure 12.1c and d).

When learning slit lamp BIO it may be difficult automatically to transpose the view into a correct drawing of the fundus. Another possibility is to draw the view through the indirect lens directly onto paper. If this is then rotated through 180° the correct orientation of the fundus features relative to each other is obtained. However, when using this method of recording it is imperative to remember that the quadrant illuminated is still the quadrant being examined, and not to transpose the drawing of, for example, the superior fundus onto the section of the recording chart designated for the inferior fundus.

Methods to assist with detecting macular oedema

It is important to be able to detect macular oedema, and Chapters 6 and 7 cover those maculopathies that should be referred for monitoring or treatment. Visualization of macular oedema is very difficult with direct ophthalmoscopy, unless the extent of the oedema is so considerable that it can be detected with monocular cues. One of the major advantages of slit lamp BIO is the stereoscopic view, which greatly assists in detecting elevation of the retina associated with oedema. In milder cases, oedema can be detected by the following procedure:

- the slit lamp beam is made into a narrow slit and focused on an adjacent area of the retina believed to be flat

- the light beam is then passed over the macula, using several slow careful sweeps
- if oedema is present the thickness of the light beam will increase in the region of oedema; hence diabetic macula oedema is referred to as retinal thickening (Kinyoun et al., 1989).

This is not easy for a novice user to observe. Sometimes a slight displacement of the light beam can help visualize retinal thickening.

It has been reported that in eyes with questionable thickening, as determined by slit lamp BIO, direct contact fundus biomicroscopy has revealed retinal thickening to be present (Kinyoun et al., 1989). The direct contact method may give better appreciation of depth, probably because reflections and aberrations are less disturbing, but contact with the cornea using this method may result in corneal abrasions.

It is important for optometrists who wish to become involved in diabetic shared care and screening for diabetic retinopathy to master slit lamp BIO, especially when this is the method of choice used in hospital departments. Several months are required to become proficient in slit lamp BIO, and the best way is to practice at every opportunity.

References

Kinyoun, J. L., Barton, F., Fisher, M. et al. (1989). Detection of diabetic macular edema. Ophthalmoscopy versus photography – Early Treatment Diabetic Retinopathy Study Report No. 5. Ophthalmology, 96, 746–51.

Chapter 13

Funding of shared care schemes within the National Health Service

William Vineall

Introduction

This chapter will offer optometrists an approach to the internecine complexities of securing funding for services in the National Health Service. It will offer a language of approach rather than a literature of NHS guide-lines and financial projections. The latter approach usually invokes weariness and cynicism amongst readers because it is a bureaucrat's preferred way of saying 'no'. The preferred emphasis on approach and ethos is intended to give optometrists a perspective on where diabetic shared care exists within the total picture of the NHS. It is likely to be more useful over a longer period if government reforms change the mechanisms and structures of the NHS, but retain the downward pressure on costs and the upward pressure on training and accreditation. The debate over which services should be provided on the NHS, and to what extent this should be based on evidence of health gain rather than past configuration of services, will continue. The strong message emerging is that health will count for more than history.

A brief summary of the structure of the NHS and its relationship to optics will be followed by a similar overview of shared care and the leading role of diabetic shared care in the expansion of clinical optometry. A snapshot of the current situation will be provided. The main body of the chapter will offer a straight-forward guide about who to speak to and how to present your arguments when approaching a Health Authority to fund a diabetic retinal screening programme. These introductory notes are important because they will enable optometrists to see diabetic shared care in its larger context: as an aspect of shared care; as a part of the increasing emphasis on primary care; and primary care's capacity to succeed in the competition for resources with all the other parts of the Health Service. It is vital that optometrists realize they are only one amongst a myriad of professions and services competing for limited resources. Any service where demand is infinite and the total expenditure is determined prior to adjudicating on those demands implies that choices must be made and that serving all demands is not straightforward. The major change since 1991 is that these choices have begun, gently, to be discussed; a user-friendly guide to diabetic shared care is but one argument within a very broad debate. Making your case for diabetic shared care is what this chapter is all about.

The structure of the NHS and its impact on eye services

The management reforms of the NHS begun in April 1991 introduced the distinction between the providers of health services (Hospital Trusts, Community Health Service

Trusts and independent practitioners) and those public sector bodies, District Health Authorities (DHAs) and Family Health Services Authorities (FHSAs), who bought (purchased) health services on behalf of central government. The major difference between DHAs and FHSAs was that the former purchased services by locally determining the contents of contracts with hospitals and community trusts (providing nursing and mental health services), whilst the latter only administered the four national contracts, originally determined in 1948 or in the case of optics 1958 and the establishment of the General Ophthalmic Service (GOS).

In 1991 optics was in the doldrums after its partial ejection from the Health Service in 1989. Ophthalmology is a small surgical speciality and, in terms of multi-million pound hospital contracts, was not of great significance. Hospitals only became Trusts gradually, and they were not fully established until 1994. DHAs had to grapple with a discipline of which they had no experience. Ensuring the books balanced and trying to establish a decent flow of information from provider to purchaser was the major concern. Radical changes in services and examination of small aspects of large contracts were not top of the agenda. DHAs were more powerful than FHSAs because they had control of more money. Moreover, DHAs were responsible for balancing their books whereas central Government was responsible for keeping the four national contracts (General Medical, Dental, Pharmaceutical and Ophthalmic Services) within their so-called 'non-cash limited budgets'. The Department of Health calculated the size of the budget, and therefore the affordable fees for each piece of work performed.

In short, optometry's profile was low in a situation where hospital costs and services were the main issue. This is not to say there was no case to be made for better use of the existing resources spent on eye care, or that diabetes was not already consuming a large amount of NHS funds. It is just that this debate was not happening.

Shared care, diabetes and primary care policy

Precisely when primary care began to develop a voice within the new internal market is hard to determine. Certainly between 1992 and 1993 there was an increasing emphasis on primary care. Part of this was due to the introduction of a management tier within FHSAs to look at how primary care services could be developed and whether they would be better integrated (this is NHS jargon for adjusting the balance of power between different groups of professionals, but raises fewer hackles) with secondary care services. Another major development was fund holding, which gave GPs some powers to buy certain hospital and community health services. Money was delegated to the practice level, but a managerial overview of how that money was spent was retained by the FHSA. The GP practice became a purchaser. Many good trees were sacrificed to the debate on fund-holding, and it acquired an unhelpful religious fervour. The Audit Commission (1996) made it clear that the reality was, like gospel truth, more ambivalent. Its report concluded that fund holding, in limited instances, had made notable improvements in service, but had been disproportionately expensive in administrative and management costs. Disciples extolled the development of service, and unbelievers bemoaned the cost and inequity of the system. Everybody was happy. More importantly but less controversially, fund holding made managers of the Health Service think about primary care, its capacity to deliver services, its convenience for patients and its possible cost-effectiveness *vis-á-vis* hospital services. Managers and clinicians began to ask if locally negotiated agreements in primary care could better address local health needs. This is where diabetes came in.

Diabetes consumes a notable part of the Health Service's budget (approximately 7 per cent of a total £38 billion budget) and affects a large number of people (2 per cent of the population or approximately 1 000 000 people, of whom only slightly less than half are identified and diagnosed diabetics). There is no readily available cure. Diabetes requires detection and monitoring. Both these tasks are expensive and involve a number of professionals who specialize in one part of the body. It is the role of the gatekeeper generalist in primary care, the general practitioner (GP), to access suitable services – podiatry, dietetics, diabeticians, optometry and specialist hospital services. It was recognized that the screening service optometrists could provide might not need to be hospital based, but would require co-ordination with the hospital and GP. Many diabetologists wished to encourage more anticipatory care in general practice, not merely responding to symptoms but pro-actively searching for complications of the disease. Retinal screening for diabetes suited this objective well.

The happy coincidence of the multidisciplinary nature of diabetes as a disease with the management emphasis on a seamless service led to an explosion of diabetic shared care schemes (49 currently). The outstanding problem remains money. Where does the funding to cover the time to dilate the pupil and examine the retina come from, when the healthcare role of the optometrist depends on the profit made from spectacle sales and the eye examination acts as a loss leader?

A straightforward answer would be that the 1997 Primary Care Act allows Health Authorities to pay for specific services at a rate determined locally. This a notable step away from national contracts determining all the activities of the optometric profession, and means that Health Authorities have some discretionary powers over primary care funding – a significant development since 1991, when optometric activity was entirely centrally controlled. It brings funding more closely into line with the managerial arrangements in place since 1996, when DHAs and FHSAs merged to create Health Authorities. Slowly but surely, the managerial arrangements in the Health Service have been unified with the purpose of looking at the needs of a local population rather than the past levels of funding required by professionals working in different parts of the Health Service. Diabetes, spanning primary, secondary and community services, is well served by the increasingly holistic view that Health Authorities are encouraged to take. Like most good legislation, the Act enshrined existing practice that responded to a general policy initiative (development of primary care) that had developed piecemeal and locally.

However, like most statements of NHS policy it leaves the disconsolate professional to reconcile encouraging words of policy with the smooth but unhelpful response of the local Health Authority, which explains that, unfortunately, on this occasion, given the severe financial circumstances and the existing prioritization of service needs . . .

Making your case

The advice and approach outlined below is intended to set the shrewd optometrist on the path to changing this depressing response. The Health Service must learn to respond more constructively to the requests made by optometrists, and still has some work to do in this field. Equally, optometrists must adapt their style and lose the assumption that, because there has been funding for GOS for many years, so axiomatically should there be funding for other optometric services. In fact since 1958, the less justification that has been required for optometry's existing status because of the existence of a national contract, the less managers have been aware of what optometric services actually cost and how they may be alternatively provided. The following section explains how to approach a Health Authority, what sort of case to make and who else to approach when working-up an application, and raises other broader issues regarding the future status of optometry as a clinical profession that ought to be clarified before approaching the Health Authority.

What is a Health Authority?

This chapter should already have made it clear that the managerial arrangements of the Health Service reflect the current Government's priorities, and therefore change not infrequently.

Optometrists must be aware that, as policy changes, so will Health Authorities emphasize different approaches for improving services.

As well as the old FPC role of pay and rations to the four family practitioner professions, Health Authorities have a general role in planning services so that the local population has the services it needs and these services demonstrably improve health. Optometrists should be aware of the current provision of services and whether they are suitable. This information is held by the Health Authority. The Department of Health sets the general policy framework for the NHS, but detailed local planning is the responsibility of the Health Authority. The Health Authority must liaise with all providers and Local Representative Committees and gather views on the suitability of local services – this is an opportunity to influence the debate.

It should be remembered that a Health Authority is not the same as a Family Practitioner Committee. Some optometrists still use this term and, just as a Health Authority manager referring to a 'high street optician' will not command respect, neither will optometrists be taken seriously if reference is made to an administrative body that disappeared 8 years ago.

Who do I speak to?

This is a problem unrecognized by Health Authority managers because the answer is thought to be obvious. In fact, it is vital that you speak to someone who has access to budgets. Do not approach the person who processes GOS claims. This is likely to be a part-time employee, or a full-time employee with many other jobs, whose role is to verify and count the GOS forms. This person will be a junior administrative grade of the finance department, and will not be a contributor to the development of primary care services. All Health Authorities have either a dedicated primary care directorate (section) or a large number of posts dedicated to working with primary care. The director usually has an obvious title such as director of primary care/

service development, but the managers within that team may be called development managers, locality managers or primary care commissioners – if you get someone called the Family Health Services (FHS) administration manager, you will have come through to the old FPC section and should ask to be redirected. A few Health Authorities have someone either partly or entirely devoted to optics, but usually the person to speak to will either cover optics along with GPs, or be responsible for all the non-GMP practitioner groups. There are a dozen Health Authorities with optometric advisers, whose role is to guide the Health Authority in its priorities for service development. You will need to speak to them too, but they only work a couple of sessions per week, and in order to get your message into the mind (and more importantly the budgetary considerations) of the Health Authority you must speak to the relevant manager. This also ensures that awareness of optometry does not disappear when the adviser is not at the Health Authority.

What do I say?

It is probably best to write a letter explaining the service you hope to set up and then follow it up with a telephone call. If you can, get the manager to visit you – it is a good way of encouraging interest in optics. You should explain why you believe the service is necessary and make it clear that you understand money is scarce and so you have developed a good service specification. Remember that funding is not automatically available and is open to negotiation. Do not dive in and ask for money at the first meeting, because it then makes it too easy for the Health Authority to dismiss your request on the simple grounds that there is no money available. This is true only in so far as there is not enough money to satisfy everyone; the skill is to persuade the purchaser that you should be satisfied ahead of others. Any good service specification must show evidence of costing, proposed training and accreditation of the optometrists involved and the establishment of an audit cycle. All of this together must allow for the demonstration of health gain.

Costs

This topic exercises people in the NHS because it is now clearer how the total NHS budget of £42 billion is spent. Health Authorities are, amongst other things, accounting units for health expenditure in a locality. The vast majority of a Health Authority's budget is accounted for in hospital contracts and votes for particular services determined by Parliament. Some Health Authorities set aside funds for primary care development, and others concentrate on transferring monies into primary care from savings in secondary care. It is from these small areas of flexibility that funding for shared care will come.

You need to be clear about the likely uptake of any service, how much time each item of service takes and what this costs you in practice. Optometrists used to the realities of a real market should be well equipped to explain how their costs have been calculated. The sophisticated optometrist could ask to see the details of secondary care contracts and calculate the price of each individual screening and then compare this with the figure in primary care. You may well come up with a strange figure, because hospitals tend to shift their overheads away from high volume services in the hope this will attract more business. The breakdown of a unit price into the service and overhead element is a calculation Health Authorities still find rather difficult to make because knowledge of individual providers' constituent costs is still poor. This is due in part to the intransigence of hospitals, because any accurate understanding of their budgets strengthens the position of purchasers. Hospitals are not keen to break down their costs, just as the Treasury has never embraced the concept of hypothecated taxes; people better understand how money is being spent and therefore can make more pertinent criticisms. A good and difficult question to ask of the Health Authority as overall planner of the service is why, if optometrists are able to provide an accurate assessment of what a service costs and must justify their service on the grounds of cost-effectiveness, cannot the Health Authority provide a similar breakdown of the comparable service in the hospital? The answer may well be that the contract has not been examined in sufficient detail (the 1991 position); if so, ask for this shortfall in knowledge to be rectified.

The rule of secondary contracting is that cost equals price, and when you are presenting your case be explicit that this is not the assumption in optometry. You should remember that all employees of a Health Authority earn a salary; issues of time and opportunity costs are not as central to managers as they are to optometrists and it is worth explaining why, without payment of some sort, an increased healthcare role is barely viable in financial terms for most optometrists. This particular issue could act as an introduction to the general issue of optometric finance; the absence of a structure of clinical payments for optometrists and the role of spectacles in the subsidy of health care. Optometrists should expect the debate to turn to whether the main professional motivation is selling of spectacles or clinical eye care. Ambivalent answers will not impress the Health Authority.

Training and accreditation

The old pattern of primary care involved taking a degree, undergoing a pre-registration year and then going out to practice without the expectation of regular retraining over working life. Postgraduate education was *ad hoc* and dependent on the ethos of professional self-improvement. There was no assumption that the demands of practice changed sufficiently quickly for further training to be required during a working lifetime. This situation has already changed markedly, and will continue to develop. Providing a particular service requires specific training, and this must be to a standard that can be tested and subsequently measured.

There has been a rapid expansion of courses on diabetic retinal screening. The best courses usually have university or hospital input, and a clear clinical standard that can be presented to purchasers as a measure of quality. Until the system of postgraduate qualifications is established by the College of Optometrists, it is best to look to the local ophthalmologist to devise a training scheme in conjunction with the Local Optometric Committee and, sometimes, the University department. It is probably best for the Local Optometric Committee (LOC) to approach the local ophthalmologist and see if he or she can offer support in terms of a training scheme. Whatever the high politics of optometry and ophthalmology, practicalities dictate that a good relationship with local ophthalmologists must be forged. Without a defined standard of clinical competence, it is very unlikely that a Health Authority will be interested in funding a new service. There is no reason for a Health Authority make an extra payment if there is no guarantee the screening will be performed any better than opportunistic screening through the GOS.

Audit

Aside from costs and training, audit is the most important aspect of any successful scheme. The NHS is very concerned with evidence-based medicine because it needs to justify the expenditure within Government by being able to show that money spent has improved health and prevented disease. This is still very difficult to do, and the issue is more established in the minds of Health Authorities than in any way solved. There is a developing policy debate about whether contracting for secondary care services is led by the business and service needs of hospitals rather than the health needs of local populations, and whether existing monies could be better spent through other Government agencies that actually do more to improve health. Only with a good amount of audited information can you hope to enter that argument and compete for resources. The GOS does not make any demands on audit because it is a nationally guaranteed sum of money, but at Health Authority level no money is guar-

anteed, so you must provide decent information.

The purpose of an audit cycle is to ensure service changes are dictated by evidence and based on data collected, then compared with a baseline prior to the commencement of service. The service must be performed to a defined standard (the training and accreditation element), and work against that standard should be monitored (data collection) and audited (data analysis) and any changes to services made accordingly. Audit is a continuous cycle rather than a single exercise. It is a big change in the ethos of primary care to monitor work that has traditionally been opportunist and responsive to symptoms. The sensitivity (the proportion of people with referable retinopathy correctly identified) and specificity (the proportion of people without the disease correctly classified) of any screening service will partly determine whether the service is funded or not; if there is no evidence that this screening programme produces sufficient benefit for a local population, it is very unlikely to be funded.

Audit is complex, requires access to good quality computers and usually needs one person working full-time to undertake data collection and entry. This is quite an investment of time and money, and you will probably need to approach the local teaching hospital or, if you do not have one nearby, the public health department of the Health Authority may be able to help. The epidemiologist may be able to give information on the prevalence of diseases locally, and some departments now have a staff member dedicated to the measurement of the incidence of diseases as they present in primary care and a list of appropriate interventions.

A member of the public health department should also be able to explain the workings of the Medical Audit Advisory Group (MAAG) which, as the name suggests, has a brief to make audit a more common part of general medical practice. The MAAG has representatives from the local hospital and medical school, and usually has a full-time co-ordinator working at the Health Authority. The group usually runs eight to ten audit projects a year, and although the majority of time is spent working on projects in general practice, diabetes, being an medical condition, falls within the purview of an MAAG. It should be possible to approach an MAAG and ask for support in auditing the optometric aspect of managing diabetes in the community.

If you begin your work with a couple of local practices, you could approach them directly and check if they have already audited their patients and have information that could be useful. The public health department may also be able to advise whether a bid could be made for Research and Development monies to fund a shared care scheme. If you do go down this route, make sure a qualified epidemiologist works on your proposal. Writing an outline proposal is relatively straightforward and optometrists, perhaps in partnership with the Health Authority manager, should be able to do this. However, without the specific training in research methods you will not be able to secure funds. These bids are considered by people predominantly from a public health rather than a health service management background. If the methodology is defective the project is very unlikely to be funded, however worthy the topic.

Representation

Optometrists are notoriously poor at representing their interests. There is a tendency to believe that discussion is vacuous and that the funding of an LOC only requires the minimum to support the costs of holding an annual general meeting. LOCs have begun to develop from their post-1989 atrophy, but professional representation should be the future goal, with a full-time officer representing a number of LOCs. All the work that goes into a retinal screening programme requires time, and it is not realistic to expect people always to meet in the evenings because it is the only convenient time for optometrists. Representatives need to be flexible enough to attend meetings at any time of the day. Crucial to establishing a wider remit and a recognized clinical role in primary eye care is the ability to convince a Health Authority that services are worth paying for. You can only do this if you are consistently seen to be persuading the Health Authority of the worth of optometry. Money is not gleaned from Health Authorities by occasionally attending a meeting to discuss a particular issue, but by consistently contacting the Health Authority and making sure it knows what your concerns are. There is a need for flexibility so that new initiatives can be quickly responded to. These are often launched following a change of focus by the Department of Health, and characteristically Health Authorities are asked to bid against a sum of money with certain schemes that they have on the shelf or are working-up with a particular group. The actual expenditure of the money is determined at a local level, and optometrists need to be as easily accessible for discussing these matters as other professions. Optometric advisers cannot do this· because they must contribute to the policy of the Health Authority and not negotiate on behalf of health professionals. It is vital that an optometric representative is seen and heard whenever primary care policy is discussed.

Professionalism

It was an underlying tenet of the NHS that, as a member of a professional group, treatment and status of each member was equal. With local contracting, discreet payments for a particular service beyond the bounds of the GOS and further training for specific services, this is no longer the case. Clinically minded as opposed to spectacle sales oriented optometrists must be prepared to distinguish themselves from their colleagues as a route to professional development and payment according to professional competence. The move towards local implementation of Health Service policy will only gather pace, and you should consider whether the contractual requirements of some of your colleagues actually serve you well. Differences are likely to emerge between practitioners, and you need to think about how you present this to the Health Authority. There is a distinct advantage in having this debate amongst yourselves and preparing a case which emphasizes that a professional standard of service requires professional rates of pay. People in Health Authorities are still not sufficiently aware of what optometrists can offer, and it must be made clear that you are asking them to pay for a type of service that could not be done better elsewhere and that you have the extra training to support this. Health Authorities need to be made aware that optometry can be a contributor to a healthier population. The upshot for optometrists is that continuing education and training must be embraced and be seen to raise standards. Diabetes, which is already a major concern to the NHS, is a useful springboard to an improved professional status for optometrists.

Optometry in the mainstream

This chapter has been authored by a generalist NHS manager, and is deliberately broad in scope. All optometrists must understand the constraints the NHS operates within – political, financial and evidence-sensitive – and consider how to respond. A commitment to clinical optometry requires an appraisal of your own and your peers' contribution to a professionalism not of reputation and past qualifications, but of service delivery and further education and training. Clarify these issues in your own mind or with a group of like-minded professionals before you begin to consider diabetes in detail.

When you approach the Health Authority, be armed with your facts and figures and be clear what you want from negotiations. The advice offered covers most eventualities and, if you make the suggested contacts, you will develop a service specification similar to others received by the local Health Authority. This is key; optometry must be seen to be in the mainstream of the NHS and aware of how the current reforms and the changes introduced in 1991 have moved the debate from the maintenance of historic patterns of service to the justification, by demonstrating their impact on people's health, of the worth of new services. Diabetes presents rich opportunities because it

demands an efficient screening service and requires better collaboration between professionals, with an increased emphasis on primary care, than has been the norm. The Government is set on measuring a successful Health Service in terms of health gain rather than the neatness of administrative structures or the continuity of professional roles. Stressing the pertinence of diabetic retinal screening to the health needs of the local population, the requirement of accredited postgraduate training and the necessity of audit to measure the success of the service will only become more important in the future.

Primary Care Groups/Trusts and clinical optometry

The Government's White Paper of December 1997 (Department of Health, 1997) both sharpened and expanded previous policy, and continued creative thinking about primary care, much to the author's relief. Whilst fundholding was jettisoned, its replacement, primary care groups (PCGs), have made the holding of some funds (be it merely for prescribing or extending to all community and some secondary care services) compulsory. The Health Authority's planning function and role in appraising health needs will become its core task, with the majority of responsibility for deciding how services should be provided ceded to PCGs and, over time, PCTs (Primary Care Trusts). Optometrists should continue to talk to the Health Authority, but start to build links with the PCG too. Shockingly to some, PCGs will have representatives of social services and nurses on their boards; professionals will speak to one another, even if they share no common language at the outset.

Optometrists should consider what services they can provide as a member or a contracted service provider of the PCG. Whilst General Ophthalmic Services will continue to be administered and paid centrally via the Health Authority, payment for diabetic and other shared care schemes, from Hospital and Community Health Services, will largely be the responsibility of the PCG, who will make budgetary recommendations to the Heath Authority. When PCGs are able to develop to PCTs, from April 2000, the Health Authority will only monitor their activity at arm's length. PCTs will be free-standing public bodies in their own right. The key message is that discussion with your PCG about the funding of shared care schemes already well established or about to begin is crucial; the general rule is that the Health Authority's discretion reduces as PCTs become better established. PCTs in particular will force professions to work more closely together and will allow for better co-ordination of primary and community services. Given that PCTs will also directly commission most hospital services, they have the potential to make shared care schemes easier to deliver.

This brave new world demands integration of professional roles where it is implied by service needs. This presages more widespread partnerships between the NHS and other government agencies wherever this will lead to improvements in health. Professional self-regulation and a new focus on clinical governance is emphasized. The importance attached to improvement of health is confirmed in the new Health Improvement Programmes (HImPs), which set out the priorities for improving health in the locality and the services that will help reach these targets. It is vital that HImPs are inclusive of all local interests, but this will require increased presence by the Local Optometric Committee when the HImP is first being developed and through its subsequent modifications. The HImP is a way of making planning more holistic, but the result of the process will always reflect in part the ability of local professionals' representatives to link expenditure to health needs and the priorities of the Health Authority and PCG. In the case of shared care, any argument will be stronger if it is clear that prior discussion with other service providers has taken place and that a bid for funds is being made on the basis of health needs and service requirements, not a narrow sectional interest. Building alliances in the new NHS is highly advisable.

Far from just providing a new set of acronyms and titles, the White Paper has quickened the pace of change. PCGs have made the voluntary local budgetary responsibility of fund holding mandatory; Health Authority's will monitor health gain, not administrative structure; PCGs (and PCTs more so) will demand professional integration and partnership; self-regulation of clinical standards will be expected and monitored; and health gain for the local population is enshrined in HImPs. Demonstrating the pertinence of retinal screening on epidemiological grounds, audit, professional improvement and appropriate qualifications are all confirmed as typical features of any decent health service. The future that this chapter tilted at has already arrived. Enthusiastic explanation that optometric involvment in the management of diabetes *already* reflects the Government's new policies is urgently required of all optometrists.

References

Audit Commission (1996). *What the Doctor Ordered? A Study of GP Fundholding.* HMSO.

Department of Health (1997). *The New NHS: Modern Dependable.* Department of Health.

Chapter 14

The East London Shared Care Scheme

Sarah L. Owens for the ELCHA Diabetic Retinopathy Screening Programme Steering Committee

Introduction

This chapter will familiarize the reader with the organization and implementation of a screening programme for diabetic retinopathy currently in progress in East London. Previous chapters have discussed the natural history of diabetic retinopathy and principles of screening, and these will not be reviewed here in detail. Rather it is hoped that the reader will achieve some insight into how this programme was initiated and its current function. Critical review of this programme will identify strengths as well as potential weaknesses. A desirable result might be modification of the programme for successful use by others.

Four factors were crucial in the inception of the East London and The City Health Authority (ELCHA) Diabetic Retinopathy Screening Programme:

1. A cohesive and capable local optometry society
2. Highly motivated local diabetologists (with previous screening experience)
3. Ophthalmologists with subspecialist expertise in diabetic retinopathy
4. Financial support from the local health authority (ELCHA).

Diabetic retinopathy is still the leading cause of blindness in the working age population (OPCS, 1990). In accordance with the St Vincent declaration, healthcare professionals were endeavouring to reduce new blindness due to diabetic retinopathy by one-third by 1997 (Anonymous, 1990). The number of diabetics in East London and The City area has been estimated at 15 000, with less than 50 per cent attending hospital clinics; therefore approximately 8000 have no formal screening. (The diverse ethnicity of East London may also contribute to social isolation and poor ascertainment by general practitioner's practices. These are, therefore, probably underestimates.) The ELCHA programme is targeting those diabetics without any form of screening.

In September 1995, financial support became available from East London and The City Health Authority (ELCHA) to fund local optometrists for services not provided by the General Optical Services. After an initial meeting of the Local Optical Committee (LOC), a proposal was put to ELCHA to fund a diabetic retinopathy screening project using fundus photography. A discussion group was formed, which included an LOC representative as well as local diabetologists, ophthalmologists and public health personnel. Initial meetings and discussions were favourable; thus the need for a successful programme was established. The first patient was screened in October 1997. The programme's success was assured by:

- involvement of local general practitioners
- involvement of local ophthalmologists for:

photographic grading of fundus images obtained by the screening optometrists prompt care and treatment of patients identified by the programme with sight-threatening diabetic retinopathy.

A Steering Committee was formed and consisted of ELCHA officers, diabetologists, a representative of the East London and The City Local Optical Society, ophthalmologists and general practitioners. This Steering Committee formulated, approved and instituted guidelines and procedures for the programme.

All optometrists in the ELCHA area were petitioned to participate in the programme. The final selection of those who participated was based on adequate coverage of the geographical area. All participating optometrists were required to attend a course conducted by ophthalmologists specializing in the care and treatment of diabetic retinopathy. The goals of the course were to:

- discuss the principles of screening
- review the clinical signs of diabetic retinopathy
- review the natural history of diabetic retinopathy
- provide instruction in patient examination using a slit lamp and indirect fundoscopy with a 90D or 78D lens
- instruct in the use and care of a non-mydriatic fundus camera (with routine use of dilating drops).

The East London and The City Health Authority devoted sufficient funds for 1 fiscal year to cover all costs of administering and conducting the programme. An ELCHA administrative officer was appointed to assist the Steering Committee in organizing the programme. The duties of the ELCHA administrative officer include:

1. Fiscal management of the programme
2. Petitioning local general practitioners to refer diabetic patients (information obtained from the general practitioner's diabetic registry)
3. Publicity:

newspaper
radio
posters for optometrists' practice windows

4. Purchase and storage of materials:

cameras
film

5. Organizing procedures for film processing
6. Printing, storage and delivery of screening forms to:

optometrists
reading centres

7. Organizing patient advocacy/translation services for the following non-English languages commonly encountered in East London and The City: Arabic; Bengali; Bosnian; Chinese; Hindi; Punjabi; Somali; Turkish; Urdu; Vietnamese
8. Implementing procedures for review of the programme by formulating and sending questionnaires to participating optometrists, general practitioners, and patients
9. Organizing meetings of the ELCHA Diabetic Retinopathy Screening Programme Steering Committee
10. Providing of finance training courses for optometrists organized by ophthalmologists.

The actual running of the ELCHA Diabetic Retinopathy Screening Programme is performed by a triumvirate of personnel: the optometrist, to examine the patient and document the fundus appearance; Reading Centre personnel, to review patient photographs and identify sight-threatening retinopathy; and database personnel, to analyze efficiency and effectiveness of the programme. The continued success of the programme is very much dependent on two other aspects. Motivation of general practitioners to review their diabetic registry and refer their diabetic patients is extremely important and cannot be over-emphasized. In addition, patient care is enhanced by the participation of ophthalmologists specializing in diabetic retinopathy, with care and treatment provided within the patient's own community.

The ELCHA Diabetic Retinopathy Screening Programme

A. Objective
To identify sight-threatening diabetic retinopathy by:

1. Dilated fundus examination by an optometrist
2. Fundus photography after dilatation
3. Review of fundus photographs by an ophthalmologist or other trained personnel.

Review of reasonable quality photographs by appropriately trained personnel would augment the screening ability of the optometrist.

B. Patient eligibility
1. The patient must reside within the ELCHA area
2. The patient must not be receiving diabetic retinopathy screening or care in hospital-based diabetic or eye clinics.

C. Patient recruitment
1. General practitioners in the ELCHA area were sent an information packet explaining concepts and procedures about the programme
2. General practitioners give the patient a referral letter to take to a participating optometrist, and indicate their own name and address on the letter as well as the patient's National Health Service number.

D. Optometric recruitment
1. Optometrists must practice within the ELCHA area
2. Optometrists must apply to and be approved by ELCHA
3. Individual optometrists (not their practices) will be registered with ELCHA

4. Optometrists must attend a training course specifically organized for and approved by ELCHA
5. Optometrists must sign a contract with ELCHA
6. Adjustments are made in the number of participating optometrists in accordance with an increased or decreased demand for screening within a particular geographical area
7. Optometrists are expected to participate in a weekly rota for use of the camera, estimated to be about four to five times per year per optometrist.

E. Optometrist procedures
1. Optometrist signs rota for week of camera use
2. The methods of patient ascertainment by the optometrist include:

   a. patient referred by the general practitioner
   b. self-referral

3. The optometrist gives the patient an appointment for a date and time when the camera will next be at the practice.
4. Examination of the patient by the optometrist includes:

   a. visual acuity with spectacles
   b. slit lamp examination (optional, but highly recommended)
   c. tonometry
   d. pupil dilatation with tropicamide 1%
   e. indirect or direct fundoscopy

5. Fundus photography using a Canon CR5 camera; four photos of each patient's fundus centered on:

   a. right macula
   b. right disc
   c. left disc
   d. left macula

6. Slides are imprinted at the time of photography by the optometrist with the following information:

   a. patient's name
   b. patient's date of birth

   c. patient's National Health Service number

   d. slide number (six digit number)

   e. date of examination

7. The optometrist informs patients that they will receive an appointment either for review with the optometrist or with the hospital, whichever is appropriate

8. If during the examination the optometrist identifies diabetic retinopathy that requires urgent care, guidelines for facilitated, urgent referral are implemented

9. A one-page form (carbonated, resulting in one original and three copies) is completed by the optometrist (Appendix A), which includes the following information:

   a. patient details including name, address, National Health Service number, telephone number, duration of diabetes, and method of diabetic control

   b. general practitioner details including name, address, and telephone number

   c. visual acuity

   d. grade of diabetic retinopathy

   e. other pathology

   f. intraocular pressure

   g. recommended action, i.e. review or refer

10. Optometrist keeps top copy of form (original) and sends copies to:

   a. patient's general practitioner

   b. Database

   c. Reading Centre with patient's photographs

11. Optometrist packs up camera for transport

12. Optometrist sends out photographs for processing

13. Optometrist reviews photographs and then mails them with accompanying forms to the appropriate Reading Centre.

F. Reading Centre procedures

1. Log in photographs, note date of receipt

2. Write in patient details on slides including patient name, date of birth, date of examination

3. Organize slides in plastic sheets

4. Review and grade slides indicating:

   a. absence or presence of diabetic retinopathy

   b. severity of diabetic retinopathy

   c. when the patient should be reviewed, as established by pre-existing guidelines (Appendix B)

   d. if referral to the hospital is required

5. Complete one-page (carbonated, one original and three copies) Reading Centre form (Appendix C)

6. Reading Centre keeps original and sends one copy of the form to each of the following:

   a. patient's general practitioner

   b. optometrist

   c. Database

7. File slides in Reading Centre

8. Complete photographic log on computer database

9. Request patient appointment at appropriate hospital for those patients identified with sight-threatening diabetic retinopathy

10. Answer general practitioner's questions regarding screening or photographic grading procedures

11. Provide feedback to optometrists regarding:

   a. photographic quality

   b. procedural problems (e.g. slide labels, incomplete forms, etc.)

12. Provide feedback to the ELCHA administrator regarding:

   a. consistently poor photographic quality (i.e. identifying optometrists who may need to retrain in use of the camera)

   b. camera problems.

G. Hospital procedures

1. Generate new patient appointments

2. Ophthalmologist to inform general practitioner and optometrist with appropriate summary of patient care and management

3. Arrange further hospital review or refer back to screening programme with optometrist as appropriate.

H. Database procedures
1. Enter data from optometrist form
2. Enter data from Reading Centre form
3. Generate reminder letter to general practitioner and patient regarding need for next review with optometrist
4. Analyse data as appropriate regarding efficiency and effectiveness of screening programme, as requested by the ELCHA administrator and Steering Group.

As this is written, The ELCHA Diabetic Retinopathy Screening Programme has just completed its first year. Reasonable success was achieved in terms of evaluating the estimated number of patients per week as well as minimizing expensive evaluation at the hospital for patients who do not have sight-threatening diabetic retinopathy. We are most grateful that the East London and City Health Authority has dedicated 100 per cent of the projected second year's budget for the continuation of this project.

Acknowledgment

The material in this chapter is based on pre-existing work composed by Mr John Bryan, representative of the East London and City Local Optical Committee. I am indebted to him for allowing me to use this material to prepare this chapter, and also for his critical review of the final product. I am also grateful to my colleagues on the Steering Committee, particularly Ms Lisa Browne, whose tireless efforts have ensured the success of this project.

References

Anonymous (1990). Diabetes care and research in Europe: the St Vincent declaration. *Diabetic* Med., **7,** 360–61.

OPCS (1990). Government Statistical Service, Office of Population Census and Surveys. *Causes of Partial Sight and Blindness in England and Wales, 1990–1991.* HMSO.

Appendix A: Diabetic Retinopathy Screening Report

This one-page form (carbonated, one original and three copies) is completed by the optometrist during the screening appointment. The upper portion contains space to enter patient details; name, date of birth, address, NHS number, etc. The middle section contains space for the optometrist's details (name and address), details of the patient's diabetic and medical history, visual acuity, and a checklist of categories of diabetic retinopathy for the screener to tick. In the fourth section the optometrist indicates the proposed recommended action for the patient. The fifth section is informed consent, which the patient signs prior to examination.

East London and The City Health Authority
and
East London and The City Local Optical Committee
Diabetic Retinopathy Screening Report

Patient Details: GP ☐   **Self Referral** ☐
Surname:_____   Sex:_____   **Ethnic Group**
First Name:_____   NHS No._____   White ☐
Address:_____   Date of Birth:_____   Black Caribbean ☐
_____   Telephone No.:_____   Black African ☐
_____   Indian ☐
Postcode:_____   Date of Appointment:_____   Pakistani ☐
General Practitioner Details: Chinese ☐
Name:_____   Date of Previous Screening: Black Other ☐
GP Address:_____   _____   Other/Not Given ☐
_____   Previous Identification No._____

Screener Details (Name & Address - Please Stamp)	General Diabetic Status Duration .... Yrs
_____	Control by Diet Hypertension ☐
_____	Tablet Pregnancy ☐
_____	Insulin
	Attending Diabetic Screening Elsewhere:
Signature of Screener	Where: _____
	Date of Last Retinal Screening Test:

Visual Assessment	**Right Eye**	**Left Eye**	If below 6/60 Please Specify Count
Best visualacuity with distance Spectacles or Pinhole	6/	6/	Figures Hand Motion or Light Perception
Near Vision	N	N	

Ophthalmoscopy and Fundal Examination after Mydriasis	Right Left	If not dilated state reason
	☐ No abnormality Detected ☐	
	☐ Fundus not adequately seen ☐	
Background Retinopathy	☐ Micraneurysms Exudates ☐	**Review in one Year**
	☐ Small Haemorrhages outside the Macula ☐	
Maculopathy	☐ Oedema and/or Exudates in Macula ☐	**Previous Treatment**
Pre-Proliferative Retinopathy	☐ Large Retinal Haems ☐	**Co-pathology/History. Please explain acuity of 6/18 or worse**
	☐ Cotton Wool Spots ☐	
	☐ Venous Beading ☐	
	☐ RMA ☐	
Proliferative Retinopathy	☐ New Vessels on Disc ☐	
	☐ New Vessels Elsewhere ☐	
Advanced Retinopathy	☐ Vitreous Haemorrhage Fibrosis ☐	
IOP	mmHg	Instrument Type
Slide Identification Nos.		

Action Recommended	None ☐ Refer ☐	**Final Action**
Comments		

Consent I,_____consent to the information on this form passed to those maintaining the Diabetic
Register and Reminder System providing it is treated with appropriate confidence by staff involved.
                    Signed _____   Date _____
White copy : GP / Pink copy with Slides: Reading Centre / Blue copy: Optometrist / Yellow copy: Central Database /Lilac Copy to HA

Appendix B1: East London and The City Health Authority Diabetic Retinopathy Screening Protocol

This chart contains a list of outcomes of screening in the left column (i.e. type of retinopathy) and the recommended action in its accompanying right column.

SCREENING PROTOCOL

1. No **diabetic retinopathy** or abnormality detected	Optometrist reviews in **12 months**
2. Background retinopathy Microaneurysms anywhere. Exudates or Haemorrhages more than one disc diameter from macular.	Optometrist reviews in **6 or 12 months**
3. Maculopathy Oedema, exudates, haemorrhages (not microaneurysms) within one disc diameter of macular.	Refer patient for ophthalmologists opinion. **Soon.** It is suggested that patients are seen by an ophthalmologist within 8 weeks of referral.
4. Pre-Proliferative Retinopathy Extensive haemorrhages, multiple cotton wool spots, venous beading/reduplication, dilated capillaries, IRMA	Refer patient for ophthalmologists opinion. **Soon.** It is suggested that patients are seen by an ophthalmologist within 8 weeks of referral.
5. Proliferative Retinopathy New vessels on disc or elsewhere. Pre-retinal haemorrhages of fibrosis	Fast Track referral for ophthalmologists opinion. **Urgent.**
6. Advanced Retinopathy Vitreous haemorrhage/fibrosis	Fast Track referral for ophthalmologists opinion. **Urgent.**
7. Inadequate Fundus View	Refer patient for ophthalmologists opinion. **Soon.**
8. Unattributable Loss of Central Vision	Refer patient for ophthalmologists opinion. **Soon**

Appendix B2: Flowchart of Diabetic Screening Procedure

This flowchart illustrates the pathway of patient incorporation into the screening programme as well as appropriate actions to be taken by all personnel involved in the screening procedure.

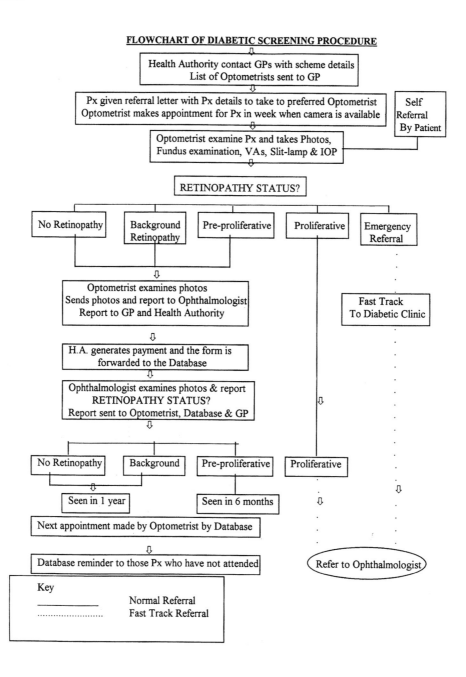

FLOWCHART OF DIABETIC SCREENING PROCEDURE

Health Authority contact GPs with scheme details
List of Optometrists sent to GP

Px given referral letter with Px details to take to preferred Optometrist
Optometrist makes appointment for Px in week when camera is available

Self Referral By Patient

Optometrist examine Px and takes Photos,
Fundus examination, VAs, Slit-lamp & IOP

RETINOPATHY STATUS?

No Retinopathy | Background Retinopathy | Pre-proliferative | Proliferative | Emergency Referral

Optometrist examines photos
Sends photos and report to Ophthalmologist
Report to GP and Health Authority

Fast Track To Diabetic Clinic

H.A. generates payment and the form is forwarded to the Database

Ophthalmologist examines photos & report
RETINOPATHY STATUS?
Report sent to Optometrist, Database & GP

No Retinopathy | Background | Pre-proliferative | Proliferative

Seen in 1 year | Seen in 6 months

Next appointment made by Optometrist by Database

Database reminder to those Px who have not attended

Refer to Ophthalmologist

Key
_____   Normal Referral
....   Fast Track Referral

Appendix C: Reading Centre report

This one-page form (carbonated, one original and three copies) is completed by the photographic grader. The upper portion contains pertinent patient details such as name, date of birth, address, NHS number, etc. The second portion contains boxes to tick as follows: checklist of features of diabetic retinopathy; checklist of recommended action (review or hospital appointment); timing of re-examination by the optometrist; and feedback regarding accuracy of the optometrist's assessment and recommended patient management.

East London and The City Health Authority
and
East London and The City Local Optical Committee

Diabetic Retinopathy Screening
Reading Centre Report

Patient Details:

Surname:_____   First Name:_____

Address:_____   Sex:_____

_____   Date of Birth_____

Postcode:_____   NHS No.:_____

Date Slides Received:_____   Screener No.:_____
Date Slides Graded:_____
Date Reports Returned to Opt etc.:_____   Slide No.:_____

Retinopathy	Right Eye		Left Eye
Unassessable/Ungradeable	☐		☐
Nil	☐		☐
Background	☐	Microaneurysms / Exudates / Small Haemorrhages	☐
Maculopathy	☐		☐
Pre-proliferative	☐	Large Haemorrhages / Cotton Wool Spots / Venous Beading / IRMA	☐
Proliferative	☐	New Vessels on Disc / New Vessels Elsewhere	☐
Advanced Retinopathy	☐	Vitreous Haemorrhage / Fibrosis	☐
Quality of Photography	☐	Good / Just Adequate / Poor/Unreliable-REPEAT ASAP	☐

Recommended Action — Hospital Appointment Made ☐ / RE-PHOTOGRAPH ASAP

Optometrist Re-examine — 1 Year ☐   6 Months ☐   3 Months ☐

Optometrist Classification — Correct ☐ / In-correct ☐   **Comments**

Optometrist Action — Correct ☐ / In-correct ☐

Reading Centre _____   Name _____ Signed _____

Hospital to retain White Copy / Pink Copy : Optometrist / Yellow Copy : GP / Blue Copy : Database;

East London and The City Health Authority Diabetic Retinopathy Screening Programme personnel:

Steering Committee:
John Anderson, Consultant Diabetologist, St. Leonard's Hospital
Lisa Browne, Dental and Optical Contracts Manager, ELCHA
John Bryan, Optometrist, East London and The City Local Optical Committee
Nicola Connor, Senior Registrar in Public Health, ELCHA
Siobhan Cooke, General Practitioner, Tower Hamlets
Sue Gelding, Consultant Diabetologist, Newham General Hospital
Zdenek Gregor, Consultant Ophthalmologist, Moorfields Eye Hospital
David Humphrey, Development Manager, ELCHA
Peter Kopelman, Consultant Diabetologist, Royal London Hospital, Whitechapel
N. Kyali, Consultant Ophthalmologist, Newham General Hospital
Ann Mackie, Consultant in Public Health, ELCHA
Sarah Owens, Associate Specialist in Ophthalmology, Moorfields Eye Hospital
Daphne Stedman, Patient Representative

Optometrists participating in the ELCHA Diabetic Retinopathy Screening Programme by area:

City and Hackney:
C. Asota
Elizabeth Devan
Robert E. Owen
G. H. Witt

Newham:
Barry Blackman
John Bryan
Angela Fletcher
Anthony Okenabirhie
Brian Roy

Tower Hamlets:
S. Brooks
Peter Croucher
Martin Hodgson
C. Longwell
John McMenemy
Philip Moss
A. Patel

Database directors:
City and Hackney:
Paul Kavanagh, Diabetic Unit, St. Leonard's Hospital

Newham:
Paul Kavanagh, Diabetic Unit, Shrewsbury Road Health Centre

Tower Hamlets:
Peter Kopelman, Consultant Diabetologist, The Royal London Hospital

Reading Centre directors:
City and Hackney:
John Anderson, Consultant Diabetologist, St. Leonard's Hospital

Newham:
N. Kayali, Consultant Ophthalmologist, Newham General Hospital

Tower Hamlets:
Sarah L. Owens, Associate Specialist in Ophthalmology, Moorfields Eye Hospital

Other ELCHA Diabetic Retinopathy Screening Programme personnel:
Sarah Ambrose-Willson, Diabetes Nurse Specialist, St. Leonard's Hospital
Val Brown, Diabetes Nurse Specialist, St. Leonard's Hospital
Jan Campbell, Diabetes Nurse Specialist, St. Leonard's Hospital
A. M. P. Hamilton, Consultant Ophthalmologist, Moorfields Eye Hospital
Phillip Hykin, Consultant Ophthalmologist, Moorfields Eye Hospital
Ann-Marie Jones, Diabetes Nurse Specialist, St. Leonard's Hospital

Chapter 15

Other retinal conditions

Peter Hamilton

While screening for diabetic retinopathy, there are other medical retinal conditions that may mimic diabetic retinopathy or give rise to referral. All patients illustrated in this chapter are diabetics. Some of the examples have accompanying fluorescein angiograms, which are very important in the differential diagnosis of retinal pathology and to demonstrate any accompanying diabetic retinopathy. One of the most common conditions that can mimic diabetic retinopathy is retinal drusen.

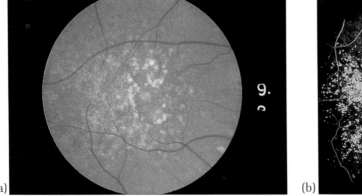
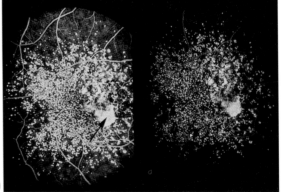

(a) (b)

Figure 15.1 (a) In this example, there are drusen and areas of retinal exudate formation. (b) On the fluorescein angiogram, it is difficult to see the retinal vascular element to this condition because of the marked hyperfluorescence of the drusen. In addition to drusen, there is also an area of pigment epithelial atrophy (arrow).

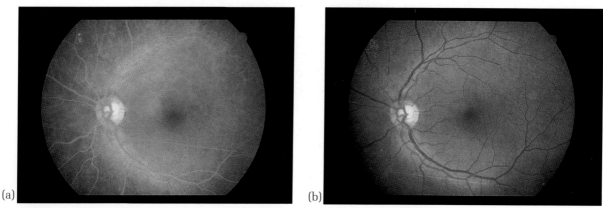

(a)
(b)

Figure 15.2 These two pictures are from a diabetic patient who had a large fatty meal prior to appearing in the clinic. (a) This shows pink vessels both on the disc and in the peripheral retina. This condition is called lipaemia retinalis, in which chylomicrons are circulating in the blood. (b) Half an hour later, the chylomicrons have cleared and the retina has taken on a normal appearance. There is no evidence of any diabetic retinopathy.

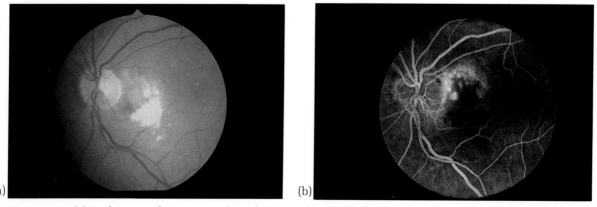

(a)
(b)

Figure 15.3 (a) In this case there are exudates between the disc and macula associated with some haemorrhages. (b) Fluorescein angiography shows a hyperfluorescent spot immediately temporal to the optic disc, and this is a peripapillary subretinal neovascular membrane.

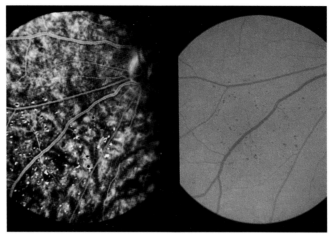

Figure 15.4 In the colour picture there are small red dots, which look like microaneurysms. The fluorescein angiogram, however, shows hyperfluorescence of these dots and the dark capping of the hyperfluorescent areas. This is very typical of a cavernous haemangioma of the retina.

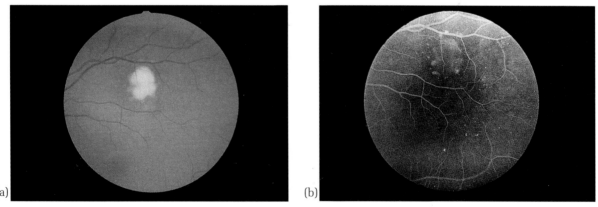

(a)   (b)

Figure 15.5 (a) This patient was referred with an exudate above the macula adjacent to the superior temporal vessels. (b) On fluorescein angiography, this exudate only vaguely fluoresced and subsequently an ultrasound confirmed the presence of an ostioma of the retina.

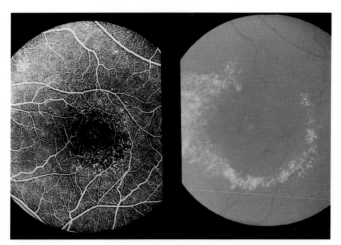

Figure 15.6 Colour picture and fluorescein angiogram showing a circinate exudate ring completely surrounding the macula in a diabetic suspected of having marked diabetic maculopathy. The fluorescein angiogram shows capillary dilatation completely surrounding the fovea and this is a case of idiopathic juxtafoveal telangectasia resulting in leakage from the capillaries and deposition of exudate.

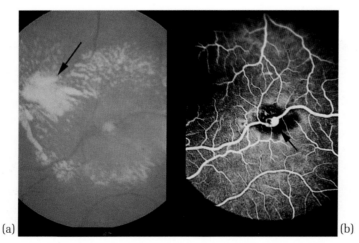

(a)   (b)

Figure 15.7 (a) This case was referred because of the marked circinate exudate formation encroaching on the macula (arrow) in the inferior temporal quadrant. (b) The fluorescein angiogram shows a macroaneurysm (arrow) as the cause of the leakage and exudate formation.

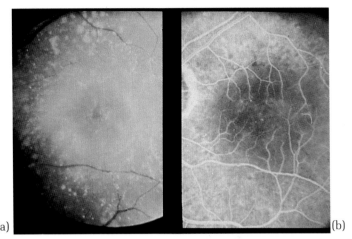

(a)   (b)

Figure 15.8 (a) This shows extensive exudate-like material across the posterior pole with an ill-defined macula. (b) The fluorescein angiogram shows hyperfluorescence of many of these exudate-like areas. This is a case of tamoxifen retinal toxicity.

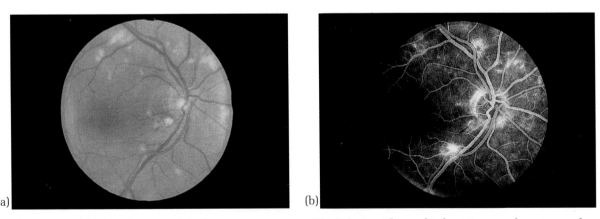

(a)   (b)

Figure 15.9 (a) This photograph is from a young man with diabetes. The multiple cotton wool spots may be indicative of rapidly developing diabetic retinopathy, hypertension or one of the auto-immune diseases such as systemic lupus erythematosus. There was no sign of any other retinopathy by fundus examination nor fluorescein angiography, and this patient ultimately tested positive for AIDS. The areas of cotton wool spots represent arteriolar occlusion as a result of precipitation of immune complexes in the arterioles. (b) On the fluorescein angiogram these areas are associated with areas of capillary non-perfusion, and in the later angiogram there is leakage from these capillaries.

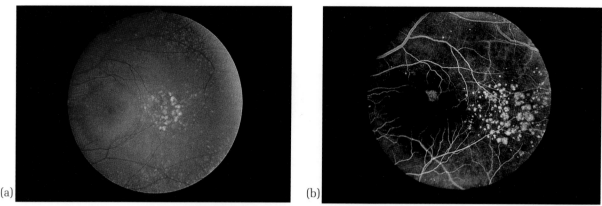

Figure 15.10 (a) The fundus photograph shows an area of exudate-like material temporal to the macula with a circular area of elevated retina. (b) On the fluorescein angiogram the area temporal to the macula shows hyperfluorescence, and in the centre of the circular area there is an area of less intense hyperfluorescence, which becomes gradually more intense in the later stages of the angiogram. This is a patient with central serous retinopathy and basal lamina drusen associated with type II membranous glomerular nephritis.

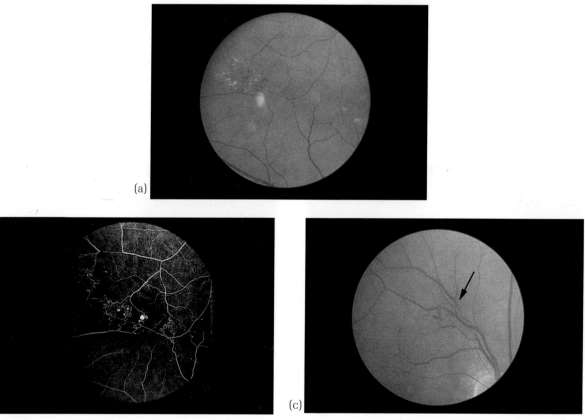

Figure 15.11 (a) This shows microaneurysms and exudates in the area immediately temporal to the macula. (b) The fluorescein angiogram in the early stages shows hyperfluorescence of the aneurysms and later leakage. Although this looks like diabetic retinopathy, if we look now at (c), the colour photograph of the optic disc area, we see that there is evidence of vein occlusion and a collateral channel surrounding the area of the occlusion. This patient therefore had a superior temporal branch vein occlusion with the blood diverting through collaterals in the area temporal to the macula.

Index